Alison's
Bits & Bobs

Alison's
Bits & Bobs

Alison x

ALISON SHATFORD

Matador
9 Priory Business Park,
Wistow Road, Kibworth Beauchamp,
Leicestershire. LE8 0RX
Tel: 0116 279 2299
Email: books@troubador.co.uk
Web: www.troubador.co.uk/matador
Twitter: @matadorbooks

ISBN 978 1838592 110

British Library Cataloguing in Publication Data.
A catalogue record for this book is available from the British Library.

Printed and bound in the UK by TJ International, Padstow, Cornwall
Typeset in 11pt Minion Pro by Troubador Publishing Ltd, Leicester, UK

Matador is an imprint of Troubador Publishing Ltd

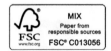

A SUNNY DAY JULY 4ᵀᴴ 1984 I HAD ARRANGED AN appointment at the doctors as I was covered in bruises and my head was hurting – as I could not walk I drove my precious Mini to the appointment (my neighbour Mr Smith had sold it to me and I named my Mini Jessica).

After having my blood test done I returned to work at Pal Wear International, Oadby and my boss Richard Brucciani asked me if I was alright and I told him of course I was. At 11.50 my boss Richard came to me to say he had received a call from my Mum and Dad Alex and Mo to say that they had received a call from the doctor to say that an ambulance was on its way to collect me from work. My knees went weak and my legs turned to jelly! When the ambulance arrived, although I was only 23 years old I could not walk to the ambulance – the whole experience felt like a complete blur and I felt like an old lady. My eyes did not feel as if they were shining blue as people said they normally did, I felt like a shadow and I felt that all the bruises on my body would be used to make a jigsaw. I had not been to hospital since I was born (I was born without a belly button as such that over the years has caused some amusement and I remember at school when I was about 11 that it caused quite a laugh in class!) I had never really liked school and although I had lots of friends there were always some bullies too! However I have got lifelong friends – we remember our Kate was killed by a car, Bay City Rollers and check trousers, Marc Bolan with his handsome smile and we all loved ABBA who got us all dancing, Elvis Presley is one person I would have love to have seen, I love to dance and love the sound of music in my ears.

Sorry back to the reason I am writing this – so many memories and life is a daily chapter to me with its ups and downs.

It didn't take long to get to the Leicester Royal Infirmary – my parents were there and there were doctors and nurses all around me and I felt very frightened. I was taken into a side ward (I think it was either Nightingale or Oliver Ward) and the next thing I remember is there was drip in my arm pumping blood through my veins. I must have slept and recall that when I woke there was another bag of blood again pumping into my veins. When I saw the doctor next I asked what was happening and he said that my blood samples were going to be sent Hammersmith hospital in London, I asked if I was going to die but in my heart I knew I wasn't – I am a fighter and this was not going to beat me in any way. I was still feeling sick and had no blood in my body – another 4 units were pumped into me, I had total faith in the medical team. The doctors have explained to me that I need to have a bone marrow test done, I was 23 years old and it was awful like a fist through a wall, laying on my side with a comforting hand holding mine – a nurse who had not attended the procedure herself before – many more bone marrow tests followed, much easier these days! Feeling a bit better but could not get out of bed as blood pressure was still too low. Who would think that the next seven years would be such a struggle – life was like a rollercoaster, in and out of hospital, home for the weekend (staying in the house and no visitors) and back to hospital on the Sunday!

I was then informed by the consultants that my bone marrow samples had to be sent to Hammersmith Hospital as an emergency – when the results came back the next day they said this had never been seen before and I had been diagnosed with Aplastic anemia! I was told that I was the 13th person in England, Wales and Scotland to be diagnosed with this! I was aware that in their own way the hospital were excited about this. Between the Leicester Royal Infirmary and the Hammersmith Hospital the doctors had to keep me safe as I was getting weaker. Aplastic anemia can be a rare and serious condition and can occur at any age. Treatment I had to have was a bone marrow transplant. The bone marrow is full of stem cells to keep the body working – red cells blood and white blood cells immune system – platelets are your clotting agent and plasma cells are white bloods which kick in if your body goes into shock, it provides you oxygen which explains my headaches – no oxygen getting to the brain.

For months earlier I had had my usually monthly periods not realising that my blood loss was much more than most women of my age. I remember a day out with my family when I had to get back to the car as soon as possible as I could not stop bleeding. My family had to get rolls of toilet paper to put in my pants, there was a hand towel in the car which proved very useful. My symptoms were extreme and I would urge any women if you start getting headaches or feel lethargic or are a women that is having a tough time with your monthly period or if you skin becomes white and your eyes are hurting (I had bruising on the back of my eyes) then please get yourself checked out at the doctors.

At this time it became clear to me as the days went by that it was not just me suffering – it was my family and friends as well. I was aware I had a strong family –mother and father, one sister and two brothers, grandma and grandpa and aunties and uncles – I knew that my mother was on occasions at breaking point and

I was not making life easy for her taking out my frustrations out on her but that unfortunately is what ill people do, they don't mean it but it happens. But despite me they all rallied round and God bless them!!

At this time the Hammersmith hospital advised that I start treatment to boost my immune system as soon as possible – drugs and more drugs, bloods and platelets daily! I was given a drug ALG (which apparently is a hormone taken from rabbits! which may explain why my visitors kept bringing me carrots and lettuce!! which gave me many hours of smiling and laughing.) However the drug did make me feel very weak and sick. As my body was being assailed with drugs I remembered all the things I wanted to do at that time whether I could or not – I wanted to smell the fresh air and the flowers in bloom, I wanted to be able to sit quietly in the park and watch the world go by and later watch the man in the moon. Would I be able to go out with the girls again my friends – we were all supposed to be going to Corfu, I should have been on that plane but as I was unable to travel I gave that holiday to my sister-in-law and I wished them all a fabulous time.

It's my birthday soon but in no position to celebrate at the moment but when I can it will be a big blowout – lots of singing and dancing!

Six months later and I am starting the second ALG treatment and the hormones are from horses – neigh! My friend Ernie has been bringing me fruits to build me up and carrots galore! He gets up early in the mornings as he has a market stall on Leicester Market and he and I had had many nights in with our friend Vera – lots of Irish music and a tipple or two.

I asked the doctor would I soon be healthy and was given the news that the drugs had not worked. Over the next seven years I still had to get the bloods and the platelets, the bloods were keeping me going but I was losing a lot of weight. The doctors

CHARITY SUMMER FÊTE
SATURDAY 15th AUGUST
2 : 00 p.m. till 5 : 00 p.m.
THE WALTER CHARLES CENTRE
WIGSTON ROAD OADBY (Opp. MOAT HOUSE)

Many Stalls - Lots to Win

Tins & Things

Tombola

New & Old

Bed of Nails

Splat The Rat

Bric 'A' Brac

Cuddly Toys

Cakes

Books

Many More

Children Have Fun
Come along in Fancy Dress
Up to 6 years old and Up to 12 years old
Competition to be judged at 3 : 00 p.m.
GRAND RAFFLE TO BE DRAWN
AT 4 : OO p.m.
TEA AND COFFEE SHOP
ALL PROCEEDS TO

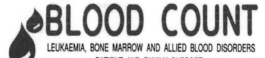

BLOOD COUNT
LEUKAEMIA, BONE MARROW AND ALLIED BLOOD DISORDERS
PATIENT AND FAMILY SUPPORT

ADMITTANCE 20p Adults Children & O.A.P. 10p

BLOOD COUNT

LEUKAEMIA, BONE MARROW AND ALLIED BLOOD DISORDERS
PATIENT AND FAMILY SUPPORT

CHARITY SUMMER FÊTE
SATURDAY 15th AUGUST
RAFFLE PRIZE WINNERS

1st	4229	J. WATERS TELEVISION	8th	5070	A. SMART SHERRY
2nd	4763	J. MORLEY GROCERIES	9th	6387	E. STANGE WINE
3rd	5185	P. WOOD MEAL FOR TWO	10th	4761	J. MORLEY WINE
4th	2065	L. LAYWOOD POT DRAGON	11th	1941	A. KHATRI CHOCOLATES
5th	1044	J. BURBETT WHISKEY	12th	3772	D. READ BISCUITS
6th	6431	J. KING TOY GORILLA	13th	3460	M. STEVENS WINE
7th	4478	V. WESTON TOY CARS	14th	4739	A. VANN TOILETRIES

THE FÊTE AND RAFFLE
MADE £ 2,050 : OO

THANK YOU FOR
YOUR SUPPORT

RAFFLE AND FÊTE
ORGANISER

Alison

MAIN OFFICE: SISTER, BONE MARROW UNIT,
LEICESTER ROYAL INFIRMARY, INFIRMARY SQUARE,
LEICESTER LE1 5WW

told me that I could go home for the weekend but I could not go out for fear of catching an infection. Mum had to tell everyone not to come to see me and my friend Tricia was a rock and helped mum with all the phone calls. At night the phone would be ringing, I never felt alone with so many people asking after me. I was happy to be home but had to take my temperature every hour. I was back on the Oliver Ward by teatime on Sunday always in a side room, the Ward Sister and her staff would sit with me and I would fall asleep and wake up in tears. Sometimes I just couldn't cope, mainly at night time but I would never let my mum see me cry.

The girls are back from the holiday to Corfu!! I would listen to all the fun stories and all the joy they had but it made me so tired and I needed to rest and it soon became that I could only have one visitor at a time.

One year later I would have to go to the hospital for routine check-ups but twice a week I would have to go to the day ward to get bloods and platelets. This continues for six years, regular trips to the Hammersmith hospital by train or car and my family would go with me. We would use the underground – I could do it with my eyes closed – Piccadilly/Central lines, I would get off the tube at the TV studio at White City and on one occasion we bumped into a tall man – Rock Hudson! We would all say that if there was no room in the hospital Wormwood Scrubs Prison would be an option on Du Caine Road. Whilst on the day ward I would take my crochet hook and wool with me and made baby clothes, hats and blankets and soon other patients were admiring my work and I was asked to make baby bonnets. I then had an idea, seeing many ladies with no hair I started to crochet hats, at this point I had no idea that I would become bald myself. It gave me so much pleasure to keep the ladies heads warm and I told them not to be embarrassed and to hold their heads high and keep their chins up. I felt I had to keep my strength up to support others, together with laugh, cry and chuckle and spent a lot of time playing games. It soon became normal to me to lie on a bed twice a week to keep my blood flowing. I thank all blood donors and platelet donors, where would we be without donors! I used to be a regular blood donor but unfortunately I can no longer do that.

Every visit to Outpatients and visits to the Hammersmith I would talk to anybody as it was a long day waiting to see doctors, blood tests and weighings. Some people hadn't got the patience but me, I learnt to be patient whether I was fit or weak, the doctors would say "you are always smiley". Conversation is very important both to listen and to talk, I do it every day. I wake up and am always thankful for the day, life is a journey and it is important to always treasure what you have got, I could always see somebody next to me who was worse than me.

As the years passed and I was home and feeling somewhat better, still not able to do anything strenuous, no partying or jogging, but I decided with the help of my family to organise a fundraising gala for the Blood Count charity which is a place at the Leicester Royal Infirmary. It was a wonderful day and the sun was shining, we had bouncy castles, bric a brac, hook a duck, ice cream van, fancy dress competition and tea and cakes. My aunties and mum must have sold hundreds of cuppas – it was an absolute hoot and all of Oadby (my home town) got involved. The pet shop gave goldfish as prizes and all the children had a wonderful time. Langmoor School also helped providing lots of games including skittles, sacks for the sack races and one family baked over 500 cakes which was a very busy stall and my old teacher Jimmy ran a book stall. I was very lucky and everyone who donated their time and raffle prizes etc said it was a pleasure to do so. Many of those involved have now passed away but it will always remain an extremely happy day in my memory and was covered by Ben Jackson of Radio Leicester who has remained a very good friend and has continued to follow my endeavours and interview me often over the last 30 years. I must mention that Oadby has continued to support me and my family to the present day. As I have said everyone had a wonderful day and we raised £2,050 which was donated to Blood Count. I can hardly believe that it had been 7 years since I was admitted to the Leicester Royal Infirmary in 1984.

My Transplant

Shortly before my 30th birthday I had a routine test at the Bone Marrow Clinic as my consultant had told me that I had one chance – a bone marrow transplant. It came as a shock as I was only given a 20% chance of survival. This was a complete turnaround in my life and I was determined that I would fight as I did not want to die and I would survive. My sister and two brothers were tested by a blood test but in the meantime I was put on the Bone Marrow Trust which is a worldwide register for finding a compatible donor/match. The Anthony Nolan Trust is a non-government funded charity which searches everyday for donors for requesters of everybody with a blood disorder that needs a life-saving transplant. I was given leaflets and information about a transplant which freaked me out and worried me. It was hurting me seeing my mum and family hurting, it was a big thing like a nightmare. I was aware that the Leicester Royal Infirmary did not have the facilities to carry out the transplant.

I was informed that unfortunately my two brothers were not eligible but thankfully my sister Annette proved to be a compatible match. Things started to move quickly with no time to waste, I was desperately ill and my sister was living in Ireland at the time with her husband Jim and four young children. I had to travel by car many times to London Hammersmith and Annette would fly over as many times as needed. My friend Tricia became a godsend helping mum and me and my cousins helped in escorting me to London. The whole family were involved as I couldn't do anything, I was so poorly and desperate for the transplant.

At this time I began for plan for the future in case I did not come home – I will tell you because it is in my heart, I planned my funeral and dealt with all my finances as I did not want to leave this burden on my family – the support I was receiving was from people who have been through traumas similar to the one I was going through. Not knowing at this time what would happen, I recall that I was out and saw a rainbow shining, I love a rainbow and stopped to watch it, it doesn't matter if you get wet, it's only water. The things we all take for granted really are the simplest, I will walk through the snow and leave my own footprints, I will see the birds in my garden and hear their songs in the early morning.

I NOW HAVE A DATE FOR MY TRANSPLANT!
– 22nd November 1991

I will travel by car with Tricia driving and my mum with me on 13th November, I went shopping with Tricia to buy easy clothing that would make it more comfortable, I got some loose jogging bottoms and button through fleece tops – I was determined that I was not going to spend all my time in hospital in a nightie – I wanted to get dressed, put on my mascara and brush my hair before it fell out! At the time I had long hair and in the time before going to the hospital I had made regular two weekly trips to the hairdresser with Tricia to have my hair cut. I knew that if I had a short haircut I would be providing hair to be made into a wig for someone else. My hairdresser was wonderful and helped me. It is a trauma for a lady or a man and chemotherapy is tough enough without the loss of your hair.

13th November was one of the hardest days of my life travelling to the Hammersmith, I had to leave my home and say goodbye to my friends and family as they waved me off. My dad had to remain at home as he has a shop – Brabazon Takeaway. Mum and Dad ran the shop and I worked in it when they would go away. The shop was a total boom in those days for the estate and the factories around the corner – cheese and onion cobs (Yummy) and turkey and stuffing cobs at Christmas. Leicester Racecourse would regularly give orders and the young lads would bring their own boxes to collect the food. Remember the bread strike? We sold one loaf at a time, the queue was long stretching from Oadby Town football club to Ellis park on the London Road. The egg scare occurred not long after but that did not stop our customers ordering their egg and cress cobs! Dad would cook roast pork and roast beef and did sliced ham. My dad is wonderful and has been wonderful and has been by my side every day, mum is soft and gentle and it took a lot of courage to stay strong as I was so poorly.

On 13th November the sky was blue and the motorway whizzed by – normal day for everyone. I couldn't focus as I was feeling worried, anxious and sad. I wanted to cry but I couldn't because of my mum Mo (my nickname for her since I was a young child). Tricia kept us going though, she put the radio on and Christmas songs were playing – will I be home for Christmas? Tricia was driving as she usually did – a little speedy! Tricia was getting married to Barnie in Cyprus and I had made sure that I arranged for her bouquet and the confetti so that she would know I was there no matter what. We had been friends for many years and I knew all the family. When Tricia got her first flat in the Summertime we decided to decorate it, we then decided we would cook a roast chicken dinner, it was a Saturday and we had worked hard all day and what is the one thing we forgot to do – defrost the chicken!! We put the chicken on the sunny window sill to thaw out, didn't really work though so we went to the chippie instead – those were the days!!

I recall that Tricia, Suzanne and friends would take it in turns to drive to the Durham Ox for nights out, we would all enjoy our dancing but years later when Tricia got married she and Barnie had many traumas as they lost their baby but happiness eventually came with the birth of Lauren Chantelle Alison was born, they named her after me because they knew I would never be able to have children of my own. I had seen a Professor Winston who had a process with test tube babies but I could not give my fertile eggs, I had missed the boat.

"Nearly there" said Tricia coming off the motorway, we found Du Cane Road. My stomach was in my mouth, I could see my mother hurting but I could not break down, I told myself that I would be back for Christmas. I just wanted to get in my room in the Dacie Ward (I had seen the room on a prior routine visit with the consultant) now I was here. Dacie Ward was a 10 bed ward for people going through a bone marrow transplant, it felt comfortable as I walked in with the doctors and nurses smiling and welcoming us. I was shown to my room which was spacious with its own bathroom. On my bed was the post – I had over 100 cards to open which was absolutely amazing – good luck cards and get well soon cards and many cards saying "you'll be home soon Alison". I was tired and weak and Tricia helped me to get undressed but there was one thing on my mind – my mum. She couldn't cope. I asked Tricia to ring my dad to come down and take mum home, I wanted mum with me but recognised it couldn't be so Tricia stayed with me overnight. I was able to have one person in my room once the treatment started, I was never on my own, Uncle Peter and Auntie Nadine stayed overnight in a guest room, Tricia would travel at weekends as she had to work. I had daily visits from Auntie Eileen and my sister's handsome husband Jim. Auntie Eileen had her own place in London and prayers were given to me each day from across Eire, Ireland. My sister phoned every day and it was lovely to speak with her and cards and letters were sent to me regularly from the children, I remember that with love now that the children are all grown up – my niece Sarah calls me "tough cookie". I was thinking of the family in Ireland – Annette had to make many trips to London for tests prior to the day, her family in Ireland were all worried not only for me but for Annette as well. She will be donating her bone marrow to me and she became strong and didn't let me worry as it was all becoming too much for me. I couldn't let myself get worried or upset or fretful as my body wouldn't be able to cope. I was so very weak, friends and family would phone me but I had to tell them I couldn't take phone calls as I was too weak but I did ask them to let them know how much I appreciated it. I slept well and woke up to be introduced to my team of doctors and nurses. Prime nurse who could answer any of my questions supported me night and day. David Marky the transplant organiser sat with me to explain the procedure. I had lots of questions to ask as I wanted to be involved throughout. I started a diary and wrote in it daily, when I couldn't do it I asked David to write it for me. He explained that a Hickman line would be filled, a Hickman line is inserted into the artery that goes into your body and carries chemotherapy drugs and the bone marrow. The next few days were very busy – blood tests hourly and being weighed. My whole body was measured by the skin – this was important as I would have to have total body radiation and it was important to target the main areas of my body where the radiation was required. David explained I would have to have three days of radiation followed by a further three days of chemotherapy. By this time only one person would be allowed in my room, the window to my room had a blind and it was closed a lot of the time for my dignity and privacy and my visitors would have phone before visiting as on many days I was too poorly for a visitor.

15th November – I was awake when they fitted the Hickman line, I watched it on the monitor as I wanted to know everything that was happening to me, it was the way that I could copy and stay strong. It wasn't easy and tear would fall on my cheek, but all I had to do was think of my family and friends. I kept telling myself I didn't want to die. Back in my room I was very tired and anything could make me feel weak, my blood pressure kept going up and down but I was told by my doctors that it was going to be 22nd November when I would get my sister's bone marrow! I was also told that my hair would fall out once I had had the radiation and chemotherapy, I started to run my fingers through my hair as it was something that worried me. I asked my prime nurse if she could shave my head before my hair began to fall out who said she couldn't do it, I was the first person to ask for this and Eddie (nurse) said he would do it Alison when the time came so later through my treatment I had comfort in knowing this would be done.

The Hickman line became sore and it was important that I had no infections. Infections would be a possible danger – I had no hope and had to sign paperwork before proceeding. Annette also had to sign and we also had to have blood tests to see if we were HIV positive which thank God we weren't because had we been I would not have been able to have the transplant. We laughed and my sister said "You'll fight girl!"

I went for radiation therapy on 16th 17th and 18th November – I was taken down by bed as I was too weak to sit in a wheelchair, Annette was with me. I had to wear a mask to avoid infections, we all had to wear masks and gowns when anyone came into my room. Once we got to the radiation room Annette was taken to a room behind a screen. The radiation room was huge and I saw a very long and narrow bed, there was nothing else in the room but high up in the viewing room I could see Annette and the radiography nurses and technicians all behind a large window screen. I had to climb on the bed, I was in fear – my life, why me? I was boxed in and couldn't move, now I know why my body screen and skin was measured, all the places where the bone marrow was needed were mainly in the breast bone, bottom of my back and hips. I had many bone marrow tests and still have dents on my body. The kindness of the two nurses was worth a million, they were caring and gave me some peace. They told me the radiation would take about two hours and then they left the room. Because I could not see anybody, I felt very lonely. They were ready to start the computer that would blast me with the radiation that I had to have, I had that treatment three times on one day!

The treatment made me feel very tired and weak and every hour a nurse would check on me. The staff at the Hammersmith were wonderful, the day and night staff looked after me round the clock. The days became so tiring and every time I dropped off to sleep a nurse would be there to take blood pressure and temperature every hour. At times I couldn't sleep because I would be thinking of mum. The radiation has now all been done so I now have to rest for three days. Later I would have chemotherapy for three days. Every night I would check my hair. The chemotherapy was full blast as I had to have every cell in my body destroyed and the full body radiation and chemotherapy took care of that. Although I became very poorly I was never sick or vomited – I was blessed and I think it must have been the prayers of my friends who were praying for me to get better. The day Annette flew home I ran my fingers through my hair and clumps of hair were in my hand – I cried and longed for my mum and Annette. Mum and Auntie Olga and Bob came down – poor dad was always driving up and down the motorway delivering family and taking them home. At the time I was having to have three baths a day, I was very weak and Auntie Olga was so strong not to break down when she was washing my hair and it fell out in the bath.

Mum was visiting me and I had been told it was a sunny day in London and I suggested she have a break, jump on a bus and go and see the Christmas lights which she thought was a good idea. She asked the other visitors whether they would fancy a short break and many agreed – I told her I would be fine – I had a mission, Eddie was on duty and I asked him if he would shave my head as he had agreed to do when the time was right. It was a joy to get rid of my hair, your hair becomes clumpy as it falls out in dribs and drabs and makes you look like a poorly hedgehog. It took an hour to shave my head and I am now bald. I had to think about mum and Auntie Olga, I knew they would have a shock when they got back, I asked David and Eddie to let them know what I had done before they came back in to see me. Mum and Olga cried when they saw me and I said don't cry, it makes it so much easier to brush my hair – which made them both smile! I was the first patient on the ward to get my head shaved and today the nurses asked the other patients if they wanted to do the same, I told them it was the best thing to do.

It is now the 20th November – two days until I get Annette's bone marrow. I was so weak that I slept a lot but wasn't in any pain except when I got an infection in the Hickman line. My body was without platelets, white cells or plasma, blood pressure was up and down and I had to drink a lot to flush away the infection. Magnesium is low. The Hickman line was very sore and they had to take the stiches out. I had decided to put a sign on my window to let family and friends know that I had no hair – TOO LATE everyone already knew!! I am very lucky to have such a long list of family and friends much too numerous to mention but they all kept me going with their good wishes.

I was very tired now as my body was struggling to deal with all the treatments but the nurses kept me laughing. They told me what beautiful blue eyes I had and asked me if I was wearing make up, not a chance I told them as I have no energy and we all laughed. My GP Dr Dadge would ring every day to check on my progress. I had received a message from Roger Morgan who had also had A Plastic Anaemia and had made a full recovery following his bone marrow transplant 6 years ago wishing me a speedy recovery. I could totally understand why he did not wish to visit Dacie Ward to say hello but it did cheer me up to hear that he was now married.

Annette flies back and checks into de luxe suite upstairs for routine pre-op checks. She spent the day with me and tomorrow is 22nd November – the day of my bone marrow transplant! Annette will be nil by mouth from midnight and I wondered how I could show her that my heart was aching, I am too poorly to have the energy to hug her and I am so tired. I did manage to sleep knowing that Annette was upstairs. I was checked every hour during the night.

It is the morning of the transplant and Annette went to the operating theatre, they were going to draw out her bone marrow at 8.00 am under general anaesthetic. As a bone marrow donor would not have any pain the hips a bone marrow puncture is not nice – I have had many. I have never been allowed to go under general anaesthetic as I could not take the risk as I had no blood products e.g. platelets that would stop the bleeding. Everyone was completely gowned up with masks, gowns, shoes etc. My room was sterilised and I could only have meals prepared in a microwave to kill any bacteria. My window blind was opened at 8.50 am and I could see David Marks, Dawn, Eddie and Eva and they were all smiling at me. My first instinct and thought was has something happened to Annette? They came into my room and told me that Annette was well, comfy and back on her ward. I was told "we have had a marvellous harvest of bone marrow cells from Annette and they were easy to draw out" I was very relieved for Annette and myself. They were excited that the operation went so well and I was told that I would be getting the bone marrow later. As Annette's blood type is different to mine (I am A positive) I was told that the blood cells would have to be rinsed out. It was a long wait, worrying and fretting with my emotions running high. Annette phoned me when she woke up and I was asleep when she came to see me but came back later. She phoned Jim and the family to let her know that she was alright and all went well (the family is very tight knitted and the strength of them all is overwhelming, they phoned me and all I wanted to do was hug and kiss them all which I will do when I am better – love is all you need when you are so poorly.

22nd November – 4.20 p.m. – the first drop of Annette's bone marrow has been transfused into my Hickman line and it was going to be successful I told myself as I want to live. Nurses checking blood pressure and temperature every hour and I was made aware that there were constant phone calls coming through asking for updates on progress. After some time the last drop of bone marrow cells have been put into my body travelling through my veins to keep every part of my body working. My body needs healthy bone marrow cells to work and save my life. I had been told that I could not get out of bed and had to use the call bell for anything I might need. I was told that the staff were going to do a carol concert at Euston Station to raise funds for the ward – I asked if I could go with them which obviously I already knew the answer to. My throat was sore and my mouth was sore and my legs were like jelly, my Hickman line had become blocked and a drug had to be used to unblock it. For the next few days it was a struggle, I could not eat or drink, my eyes became sore and my body felt shattered, it made me finally realise what I had been through!

The day came when Annette had to return home to her family, I was going to miss her so much but she said she would ring me every day – which she did three times a day, I love her so much!!

My Hickman line is getting very sore again but I continue to stay positive.

Four things happened on 22nd November that year – my transplant, the Croatian war broke out, Freddie Mercury had passed away and Gary Lineker's little baby boy was born and he was diagnosed with leukemia at 8 weeks old.

Day 10 – Monday 2nd December. I have managed to make my own bed, I have also managed to spread a round of toast and eaten a packet of cheese and onion crisps which I could taste! Also my Hickman line has been removed – what a relief, all of my antibodies, bone marrow and platelets have used this line – I called it the "Hickey line" as it has been as busy as the Piccadilly line on the underground. I have told everyone that I am keeping a diary about my transplant and asked them if I am unable to write it up will they help me and they have all said of course we will.

(I have kept in touch with a lady called Petrina and she is Malaysian and she was a donor for her brother. Petrina has travelled to England and was staying until her brother was well enough to return home.)

I have been told by David Marks that there is an injection that can be given to me to help my recovery, apparently it is expensive and the decision has to be made by the Board. I am fortunate enough that the Board members have approved the expense – I am very happy and it means a million to me.

When I first went into hospital I took with me my Mickey Mouse toy that I had purchased when I went on holiday to Florida with my friend Jo, it was the first time I had been on a plane, we flew with Freddie Laker and it was a jumbo jet – I think during that holiday I must have had some signs that I was becoming unwell as I was very weak and suffered very heavy bleeding on my period whilst walking to Disneyworld. I decided when I was going for the injection that I would take Mickey down with me so I wrapped him in the sheet on my bed. However, when I got back to my room Mickey was gone, I was very upset but the staff on the Dacie ward said they would check the laundry. It was an anxious time but the next morning my window blind opened and everyone was smiling – Mickey was back! He had been up the motorway, been through the washing machine and the dryer – I couldn't believe it but he was back.

The staff had done the carol service and it had gone very well they told me.

Day 13 – I woke up feeling much better, I bathed, dressed and put on mascara, eyeliner and lip gloss. My phone calls keep coming which keeps my spirits up. I had a go on the exercise machine – I am jiggered now. Dawn and the nursing team came to me and told me with excitement that I had a white blood count of 1.4 –WOW!!!!! They arranged a water bed for me which although felt a little strange to start with, I felt like a queen. So special, I am getting the best treatment and the news that my white blood count and bone marrow cells are going up the ladder was absolutely wonderful.

Dawn came to take my temperature but I had just had a cuppa soup so Dawn sat on my bed and said "I'll have to stick it up your bum then" – we both laughed. She gave me another one of the tablets I have to take which has a really nasty taste

– yuk. Time for my next injection in my tummy which is now looking like a pin cushion. I was also told that I will be using Annette's blood group for the next three months until I start making my own. One thing I could worry about is GVHD (Graft Versus Host Disease). It is very important therefore that I start to make my own blood but unfortunately it is a waiting game. I have given my consent for my body to be used as part of any research , Jill Howes is working at Bristol Hospital as a researcher and she has thanked me for giving my consent and over the years my bone marrow tests and healthy blood counts have been used.

It is now day 18 10th December 1991. David has explained to me that there will be a further 82 days to get by so with positivity, courage and strength I will get through. All the tests were performed daily and no sign of GVHD. It is looking very good. David explains that when I go home I will have to take my temperature 4 times a day and when I go home I have to phone him not the LRI or the GP. I am to be referred to a Gynaecologist Mr Alaziwi at the LRI 3 months after my transplant as I have had total radiation and chemotherapy. I won't have any hormones now. David has told me that he knows I am sensible and I have to have a list of all my medications with me at all times. A total of 58 different tablets for 3 months when I get home.

Mum and Dad are vistiting – another sack of cards and letters to read! Mum is coping well thanks to family and friends, Annette and Jim have sent me a video of their children, my nieces and nephews which is cheering me up no end as I love them dearly. All the teams are very excited as am I – my counts are going up sky high, another very good sign. David is looking to get me home now, four weeks to the day I arrived and I had been told I would be here for 12 to 15 weeks. Before I came to hospital I had given Mum some money to get all the carpets changed, she says they look lovely, and I am now going to have a chance to see them for myself as I have been told I can go home once the dust has settled from the fitting of the carpets, it is unbelievable after only 4 weeks. I have had a bone marrow transplant and my sister says that she would do it all over again if necessary – no worse than having a blood test.

David has given a list of all the medications I have to take around the clock 24/7. Granted I will not be able to go out but at least I am home. I will, however, have to travel back to the Hammersmith every week for 3 months. I had to get a chart and write all the medications on it, it is important to take all the meds, the most important of which will be Cyclosporine which is used to prevent organ rejection, all people who have had transplants have to take this as my body could yet reject my bone marrow. However, I now have my own blood count. I was told that when I attend at Outpatients not to take the Cyclosporine.

Mum had asked Uncle Maurice and Auntie Mavis if I could stay with them for a short time while the carpet dust at home settled and they were delighted to do so. The day finally came and I am leaving hospital – washed and dressed, eyeliner and mascara in place, I look like a balloon from all the medications I had to take but it doesn't matter to me at all. I asked if I could go and see the Christmas lights knowing full well that I could not but I promised myself there and then that one day I would see them in all their splendour. Uncle Maurice loved having me stay with them, he is Mum's brother and I loved listening to all his stories, Auntie Mavis is a choir singer and keeps busy running the church and doing the church flowers. Uncle Maurice told me about their caravan in Backton and says he will take me there when I can travel. I was comfortable staying there but at the same time really wanted to get back home to Oadby. Mum rang every day, I was there for just over a week then I got to go home to my beloved Oadby. As we drove home

I could see Brabazon Road ahead of me – I never thought I would see this again. It was getting dark and the houses had their Christmas lights on. Our home is above the shop, a large flat where we all grew up, there were 18 stairs to reach the flat and I had to lie down on my bed when I got there. The house phone is ringing constantly – family and friends all sending their further good wishes. My home looked great with all the new carpets installed. I slept for 8 hours, I felt quite weak but many thoughts were going round in my head. I had so much to catch up with in the outside world – my neighbours, friends and my boss Richard. Every time I dozed off Mum had set an alarm clock to remind me to take my medications. Mum would be there with a pint of water to help me take my tablets, it was very daunting and made me feel sick every time but I knew it was essential.

For the next four weeks I had to travel to London for check-ups, David told me on one occasion that I no longer had to take the Cyclosporine – this meant that my body was not rejecting the bone marrow – it is looking good for me!! I was also told that I could now go out in public, I couldn't believe it. Although my hair is showing signs of growing back I still had to wear a mask and a woolly hat.

I then received some bad news, my dear friend Janet had passed away, she had been ill for a long time and it was a shock for me and I wanted to go to her funeral. The day came and I walked to St Peter's Church, I saw everybody from the village as Janet was very well known. I grew up with her and all of her family, from Sandhurst Street Infant School all the way up to Beauchamp College and I remember that Janet and I always looked forward to Fridays as on the way to Sandhurst Street the lollipop lady would always have sugar coated lollipops on the wall and we were allowed to pick which colour we wanted. Those were indeed the days.

Around this time my friend June came to see me with her daughter, I found out the hard way that coming into contact with chicken pox can be harmful to transplant patients and I had to spend 3 days at the LRI. Obviously June was not aware at that time that her daughter was not feeling well or she would never have brought her round. As children June and I lived 7 houses apart and used to take

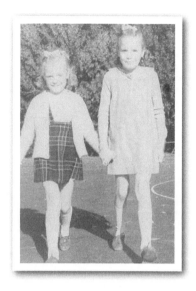

turns playing at each other's house – which was made somewhat difficult as in between there lived a dog called Max who used to chase the children as they walked past. On one occasion I was on my way to June's house after buying my dolly mixtures from the shop and when Max chased me I recall dropping all my sweets on the road – I was not happy. Mum had rung June's mum to say I was on my way and June's mum took Max back to his own house and asked the owner to keep him indoors as he was scaring all the children.

My hair is now growing back and although some patients have different coloured hair following a transplant I am pleased to say that mine remained the same colour – blonde. I recall that Annette and I had had a photo shoot at Langmoor School and the night before Mum had put pipe cleaners in our hair so that it was curly for the photos.

My strength is also coming back, there are less visits to the Hammersmith, less medication to take. I now referred to go back to the LRI where the Haematology department looked after me and they still do.

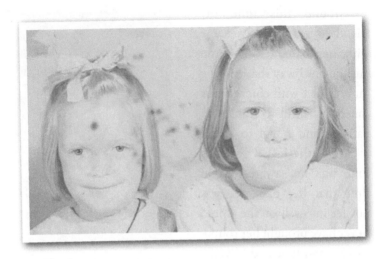

I returned back to work 6 months after my transplant, it was good to be back and Richard was pleased. He had kept in touch with Mum and Dad and offered any help that he could give. I was given light duties and all the staff were delighted to have me back. Friends were great and always there for me.

After the New Year I had a setback. In February I had pneumonia and I was back in the LRI, I was very poorly and in pain. I was given morphine and it was the only time I wasn't in control of my body. My family were called in as it was taking its toll on me but someone was looking after me and I did recover.

After I came home I decided I would never look back again – I would talk about bone marrow transplants and try to help those facing a tough time and fundraise to raise awareness. It is not only the patient who is affected but also their family and friends. I only take medications for my transplant now – penicillin each day for life and hormone replacement. I put all my strength into whatever I do as I can remember a time when I couldn't walk, climb stairs or run. I can now drive my car again and my life is starting to get back on track. I decided to change my job (I had worked for Richard at Pal Wear International for 11 years) and Richard and

Sheila applauded my decision. I saw an advert in the local paper for a receptionist at Bishop & Bishop, I made the phone call on the Saturday spoke to Derek Slater who liked my telephone manner and he rang me back on the Monday and offered me the job – WOW!

—

Before I started my new job, I was told by the doctor that I could go to visit my sister Annette in Ireland as St James Hospital in Dublin had a bone marrow unit so if I had any complications whilst visiting I could go there. I packed my bags and couldn't wait – I was going to see Annette, Jim, Michael and Katie. Jim is a wonderful husband and father but he had had his own traumatic time. He was in a car crash and was given the last rites at the roadside. Annette had not told me this when I was in hospital as she didn't want me to worry and wanted me to concentrate on getting better. Thankfully Jim has made a full recovery and is so proud of his family who have supported him as I do.

I arrive in Eire – what a greeting, all smiles and hugs. I stayed with Annette for two weeks and it was wonderful. I told them I would be back at Christmas as Christmas is a time for children – the family was growing it was now Michael, Katie,Sarah and Christopher. I would ship out and post Christmas presents every year – yellow teasets, drum sets, toys, stories and games – you name it I have sent it!

Back home now and I loved working for Bishop & Bishop and I love the customer side of the job, I am a people person and always have been. John Bishop soon became my second boss, I brought a bike for work and sailed down the Wigston Road in the Summer and drove my car in the Winter. Staff became good friends and we would enjoy skittle nights at the pub across the road The Star & Garter and we would go for Christmas parties too. The mechanics would look after my car which was an Escort Mk 3, I then graduated to an Escort Mk 4 which I also named Jessica. I now own a Mini of which I am very proud. I worked for Bishop & Bishop for 7 years as a receptionist but before I left Bishop & Bishop I had a routine visit to the LRI and then it soon became 1 year appointments at the Hammersmith.

I then became a carer as I wanted to help the elderly in their homes. As a carer I could give my time and it was a total hoot, all my clients knew that they could trust me. We would have a cuppa and a slice of cake after I had finished my chores, I love housework and respected the homes I visited.

Mum's 60th Birthday, 1998

I T IS NEARLY MUM'S 60TH BIRTHDAY AND WE HAVE TO celebrate. She has brought up four children two boys and two girls with all the ups and downs and tears and joys. Mum at this stage had 8 grandchildren and to see her love for all of them is a joy. I still have a brass bell on my fireplace that was mum's which the children used to ring until Mo would say "that's enough", she would tease them and chase them round the room.

One day we became concerned because mum had developed a nasty cough. She has had many trips to the doctor and eventually a hospital appointment. Tests began and there were regular visits to the hospital. We started to plan her 60th, had a lovely cake made and arranged visits from all the family, her brothers and sisters who all wanted to make sure that Mo had a lovely day. On her actual birthday (19th March) we had to go to the hospital so that mum could get her results, she was told that she had lung cancer – this was a shock and I just wanted to wrap her in cotton wool. We returned home and had a glass of bubbly and cut the birthday cake, we shut out the visit to the hospital – it was a lovely day all things considered. Life is so cruel in so many ways, she had to have an operation to remove the cancer from her lungs. We waited and waited at the hospital for mum to get back to the ward, when she came back I thought she looked beautiful. However the doctor told me and dad that the operation could not take place as the cancer was too close to the other organs to remove it – we were in shock and thinking how we could tell mum. Dad was devastated. I had to phone Annette and Uncle Maurice who let the family know. Mum woke up and had a cup of tea and the doctor told her the sad news. Mum's courage was amazing, she decided not to have radiotherapy or chemotherapy as she had seen what I went through. Mum came home and was fitted with an oxygen mask to help her breath. All mum wanted was her family and the children around her and whilst she was in hospital I would go to work and dad would open the shop and our friend Ann would help out. My boss at Bishop & Bishop was very kind and understanding. When I finished work I would cook a meal for dad and then drive to the hospital but on the way I would stop at the chippie and take mum in fish and chips – the other patients loved this and for the next two weeks they would all have fish and chips and when the night staff came in they would have chip butties – the ward smelt like a chipshop! Mum loved the laughs and banter and would make the nurses laugh. One day a voice chirped up "anybody got any salt and pepper?" and I said would bring some in the next evening which I did.

I did all I could to make mum smile, I can't lose mum but I noticed she became weaker, what do I do I thought, it hurts. Everyone has a mum – love her and never stop loving her. I would sit with mum playing card, mum liked to do dot to dot and colour with wax crayons (she always had a bucket of crayons for the children). She also liked her raspberry rippers, Frys cream and boiled sweets. I would cook her scrambled eggs on toast but

I soon noticed that it was becoming smaller portions as she was getting weaker. Maurice her brother would visit and lie on the bed next to mum and reminisce about the old times. Maurice was the rock of the family, he had five sisters and two brother and was a cook in the Navy.

Mum was always so tired now and spent all of her time in bed. She did not actually get out of bed again, it saddens me to have to say that in the January I lost my dear mum Mo. The two weeks prior to her passing were a blur and I have blocked it out. She was so loved by all and she would be proud of me today, I know that for sure. I have been told that I am psychic, I have had many things happen to me and that I have an aura around me, I feel mum is with me every day. Grandad Mayes had a feeling that I would become poorly but he passed away just before I became ill but I have felt his presence around me on many occasions. As they lived on the same road as me I would visit Grandma Mayes every day after work.

As time went by after losing mum, I felt very lonely and one day I said to dad "can I get a cat?" I wanted a long haired black and white male cat so we went to a lady who lived in Great Glen who looks after strays and rescued cats. There were many cats there but one cage was drawing me to it, the cat came up to the front and I said "That's Jack!" I took him home and he gave me so much love and comfort and made me want to smile. Jack was also a great comfort to dad when I went back to work, dad was really missing mum as they had been together since I was 13 years old.

One day at work my boss John Bishop called me into his office, he had a tray of tea and biscuits and sat me down and said "Alison, I want to give you a holiday". My mouth fell open and I was lost for words (which for anyone who knows me is a very rare occurrence!!) He said I don't know anyone who has been through as much as you have – first your transplant and then sadly losing your mum. He put the vouchers on the table and told me to book a holiday and I did as I was told. I rang my sister to give the news of what my boss had done for me and then rang dad to ask if he would be alright looking after Jack. I went into Going Places in Oadby and asked where I could go on my own. With their assistance I found a lovely 10 day break to Ca'n Picafort in Majorca – my holiday was booked and I could hardly wait! I spoke again with my sister admitting to her that I was a little nervous and apprehensive about travelling on my own and her response was simple – she said Alison, if anyone can do it, it is you!

On finding out that I was going to Ca'n Picafort my friend Tony who worked at the Royal British Legion in Oadby asked if I could take a gift to friends of his who owned a bar there. Of course I said yes assuming that it would be possibly a book or a box of chocolates but I was totally unprepared for being presented with a 7 foot cardboard cut-out of John Smith holding a pint of beer, thankfully it fitted into my suitcase. I arrived at my destination and the hotel was fabulous with very friendly people. Once settled in my room, I decided to go in search of the London Bar with John Smith by my side. Once I located the London Bar I was greeted by Manola and Alex, I introduced myself to them and explained I was a friend of Tony and Gill from Oadby. I then presented them with their present and said "a gift from Tony". Manola could not resist getting the camera out. While I was there, they both looked after me, showing me around the sights and made me very welcome.

On my return I was aware that dad was still feeling lonely without mum even though Jack was there and I was aware that he had not really been out socially since mum died. I suggested we went out for a drink and took him to the local Weatherspoons when I had many friends. I introduced him to everyone I knew especially the men who were of his own age. This became quite a regular occurrence and eventually he and his friend John started going out on a Friday and Saturday night for a few pints or more.

BEN NEVIS SUMMIT 4,408ft
PHOTOGRAPHED AT BRITAIN'S HIGHEST POINT

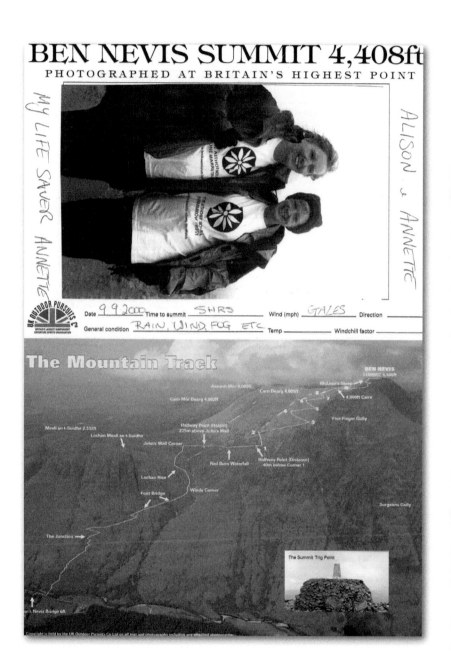

MY LIFE SAVER ANNETTE

ALISON & ANNETTE

UK OUTDOOR PURSUITS
BRITAIN'S LARGEST INDEPENDENT
ADVENTURE SPORTS ORGANISATION

Date 9.9.2000   Time to summit 5HRS   Wind (mph) GALES   Direction _____

General condition RAIN, WIND, FOG ETC   Temp _____   Windchill factor _____

The Mountain Track

BEN NEVIS
SUMMIT 4,400ft

Aonach Mor 4,005ft

Carn Mor Dearg 4,002ft

Carn Dearg 4,005ft

McLean's Steep

4,000ft Cairn

Five Finger Gully

Meall an t-Suidhe 2,332ft

Halfway Point (Height)
275m above John's Wall

Lochan Meall an t-Suidhe

John's Wall Corner

Red Burn Waterfall

Halfway Point (Distance)
40m below Corner 1

Lochan Rise

Foot Bridge

Windy Corner

Surgeons Gully

The Junction

The Summit Trig Point

...an's Nevis Bridge 6ft

Copyright is held by the UK Outdoor Pursuits Co Ltd on all text and photographs including any attached photographs

33

SOME SNIPPETS OF INFORMATION ABOUT
BEN NEVIS, BRITAIN'S HIGHEST MOUNTAIN

FIRST, THE NAME
Ben Nevis is almost always referred to by climbers as simply The Ben. Nevis is derived from the Irish words "neamheis " meaning terrible and another Irish word "ni-mhaise " meaning no beauty. However the first detailed map of the Scottish highlands draw by Timothy Pont in 1595, shows the mountain as "Bin Novesh "

THE MOUNTAIN TRACK

Ians Nevis Bridge to Junction	660m	Junction to Windy Corner	1025m
Windy Corner to Lochan Rise base	502m	Lochan Rise	137m
Lochan Rise top to John's Wall Corner	552m	John's wall Corner to Red Burn	553m
Red Burn to Corner 1	404m	Corner 1 to Corner 2	330m
Corner 2 to Corner 3	540m	Corner 3 to Corner 4	267m
Corner 4 to Corner 5	244m	Corner 5 to Corner 6	267m
Corner 6 to Corner 7	178m	Corner 7 to Corner 8	167m
Corner 8 to 4,000ft cairn	66m	4,000ft cairn to McLeans Steep	748m
McLeans Steep to Summit	526m	**Total 7.16K (4.45miles)**	

Survey by Logistics and Technical Support Dept, UK Outdoor Pursuits Co. August 95

THE HEIGHT OF BEN NEVIS
There is great controversy regarding the true height of Ben Nevis, so lets set the record straight. The 1794 map of Scotland proclaimed, "Ben Nevis is, at 4370 ft the highest mountain in Great Britain", although it should be remembered that this new map was simply an updated version of the 1782 map drawn by Lt. Campbell. By 'updated' it is meant that this was the first map showing the summit of Ben Nevis as Britain's highest point, prior to this it had been accepted that the Cairngorm area held this claim to fame.
Many people (and many reference books) still give the incorrect height of 4406ft. The postwar triangulation of 1964 gave the new height of 4418ft. But, and this is the main point, this height was that of the Flush Bracket at the base Survey Levelling Plate built in to the base of the Triangulation pillar and NOT of the ground height. As the pillar on the cairn is nine and a half feet high this makes the actual ground height 4408ft and 6". Mountain heights are by tradition rounded down so the true height of Ben Nevis is 4,408 ft. All mountain heights in Britain are calculated from their altitude above Ordnance Datum which is the average elevation of the sea at Newlyn in Cornwall.

THE SUMMIT OF BEN NEVIS - THE TRIG POINT.
On the summit of Nevis next to the ruins of the observatory you will find the Triangulation Pillar. This is more often than not simply called the Trig Point. [Grid reference 166(5) / 712(8)] Many experienced climbers and walkers will tell anyone who will listen that Trig Points are always found at the highest point on a hill or mountain. This is incorrect. They are actually sited so they can be seen from the surrounding hills, in many cases this is the highest point, but not always. It is important that they are positioned in this manner as each Trig Point forms a corner of a triangle, polygon or other geometric shape. This is used to produce an accurate framework which in turn is used to provide very exact fixings to the latitude and longitude, thus allowing the map maker and others to be able to work out their precise location anywhere in Britain.

THE SUMMIT OF BEN NEVIS - OBSERVATORY AND HOTEL
The footpath and observatory were both constructed during the summer of 1883. The contractor was James McLean of Fort William. The last rise on to the summit is named McLeans Steep in his honour. The observatory although formally opened on Wednesday October 17th 1883 did not start operating until November 28th. The observatory was built to record "The diversity of the mountain environment" eg. temperature, wind speed rainfall, air pressure etc. During 1902 it became apparent that insufficient funds were available to continue the running of the observatory and it was closed on October 1st 1904. Although one room, of the keepers hostel, was opened during the summer months as a small refreshment room. This continued until 1916. The observatory fell into disrepair, this process being helped by a fire during 1932 and the actions of both weather and unthinking climbers.
Some time after the observatory started operating, a Fort William hotelier opened a small hostel/hotel connected to the main building, this was run by two local ladies on his behalf. This hotel continued receiving guests right up until the end of the First World War. There were four bedrooms available at ten shillings per person, dinner, bed and breakfast.

LONG JOHN AND A WEE DRAM ?
No work concerning Ben Nevis would be complete without at least a mention of The Ben Nevis Distillery. Long John whisky has been produced at the base of Ben Nevis since 1825. Still bearing the name of it's founder Long John MacDonald. Long John was a direct descendent of John MacDonald, Lord of The Isles, who in the late 1300's, who was married to Princess Margaret the granddaughter of Robert the Bruce. Long John was born in 1798 and in 1825 built the first legal distillery in the Fort William area. Queen Victoria was so impressed with his "cratur " that she had a full cask sent to Buckingham Palace after her visit to Fort William. The Gaelic for whisky is "uisge beatha " meaning water of life.

* Triangulation and heighting information kindly supplied by Ordinance Survey.

Published by  28 Upper Dicconson Street,
Wigan, Gtr. Manchester. WN1 2AG.
Tel: (01942) 826256   Fax: (01942) 829579

By this time the shop was closed and the upstairs flat became too big for just the two of us. Many a day mum had said she wanted a bungalow but unfortunately this never happened for her. Dad and I decided to sell the flat – no more 18 steps to climb and we moved into a lovely bungalow on Foxhunter Drive, I had always wanted a bay window, a back door and an outside tap. The garden is beautiful with all the trees and flowers and shrubs, garden shed and pond. It had everything even my own parking on the drive – it was a dream. Everyone takes these things for granted and now they were mine.

My hospital appointments were becoming less and less, by now I realised that I wanted to be helpful to others and started fundraising and appealing for bone marrow donors to join the register. The Anthony Nolan Trust gets absolutely no Government funding and relies solely upon public donations, for people who have no faith in the Trust, I am living proof that bone marrow transplants do work. As part of my fundraising I had decided that I would make my first event climbing Ben Nevis in May 2000 and Annette agreed to do this with me. Somehow Central News found out about the climb and I was at work when I received a phone call from them asking if they could come and interview me. I asked my boss if I could leave early and when I arrived home there were four TV crews waiting for me – Central News, BBC News, Ceefax and Ntl News. The interviews went out on the same day and were repeated each day – due to the news coverage so many people contacted saying well done Alison and asked if they could join us on the walk up Ben Nevis. JR Camping of Lee Circle, Leicester gave myself and Annette all the walking kit, jackets and fleeces that we would need. Annette flew over from Eire and joined me at the railway station in Scotland and with a bus load of happy people we travelled to the hostel in Ben Nevis. We soon all got to know each other and many of the others had a connection for whom they were making the climb and wanted to join the appeal for the Anthony Nolan Trust. Ben Nevis was hard work, we had rain, storms and sunshine, halfway up the climb we had to be roped together and when the clouds met our faces there were runny noses, red cheeks and cold hands – the waterproofs were essential. It was also hot walking and on occasions we had to remove some clothing. My friends John and Sandra joined us on the trip although only John made the climb while Sandra watched from the ground. We were all delighted to have reached hallway up – make no mistake Ben Nevis is not a walk it is a climb. Some of the rocks were enormous and there were times when I had to go up on my bum, John helped Annette but we enjoyed it all. The organisers were great, I would ask are we nearly there yet? Round the corner they said but there were so many corners! From start to finish in total we climber 4,408 feet. Soon there was joy we were only a short way from the summit. The clouds were coming down fast as we were reaching the summit and wow what a feeling when we reached our goal. We all hugged each other and as I hugged Annette I said "we did it" and then gathered for a group photo. The clouds were now thick and foggy as we started our descent, it was tough with the large rocks and steep steps. It took 5 hours to get to the top and 3 hours to get down. I felt great and my health was amazing, to think it was only 5 years ago I had no strength and I have now climbed Ben Nevis. It was now party time and it didn't matter to anyone that we now felt jiggered, we had a great meal and danced all night long – party, party, party!! A few drinks later we were all treated to a hot toddy compliments of our hosts and Annette asked "What are we going to next Al?"

The next morning we all boarded our coaches to the railway station and Annette left to get her flight home. We all departed together and everyone was happy, those people who had contacted me lived up and down the country, it was an absolute pleasure to meet everyone and I thanked them all for answering my appeal for bone marrow donors and funding. I raised £3,007.60 and since I started the total is now an amazing £3,677.60. I continued to appeal for donors and raising awareness of the need for bone marrow, it is something that we don't think about and I know that everyday someone, somewhere is going to need a donor and I feel so lucky that Annette was a compatible donor.

Over the years we have organised raffles, auctions, been to all the shops and pubs in Oadby shaking donation buckets, all the shops and businesses have been great providing donations to the raffles and auctions, Leicester City Football Club have sent signed shirts and footballs, Gary Lineker sent me a Match of the Day script for the coverage of the final of the World Cup, Tigers Rugby had also provided shirts etc towards the raffles and auctions, Oadby British Legion were also involved as was the Oadby Working Men's Club (which sadly is no longer there) got involved. I held my 10th anniversary celebration at the working men's club – those were the days. At this stage I have raised over £10,000 for the Anthony Nolan Trust. This is most rewarding but it remains the fact that it is all about raising awareness and encouraging young adults to join the bone marrow register. People have been so generous in donating things such as Easter eggs, Wendy houses and knitted socks for the walk to Ben Nevis.

Next challenge with Annette – we went to Spain – a pilgrimage to the Santiago de Compostela and Annette started her own fundraising for lukemia and St James Hospital in Dublin. The fundraising group had set the event and Annette asked if I would walk it with her and of course I said yes. I decided that I would raise funds for Anthony Nolan and also the Irish bone Marrow Trust, I raised £750 and I donated

£1,000 euros to Eire. I flew to Dublin to meet Annette and 30 more people, it was a pleasure to meet them as they knew me through Annette and had always prayed for me. We met at the Arthur Guinness Co. Ltd on 17th August 2002. Once we arrived in Spain we would be walking for 10 days at 30 kilometres a day, I remarked to Annette that it would be warmer than Ben Nevis and indeed it was, it was hot very hot, plenty of sun cream needed and I never go out without it as I have had chemotherapy and radiation therapy.

The pilgrims walk was great taking in all the wonderful sights, sun shining and the beautiful blue skies with no rain or wind. It was amazing, smiles all around. Our organisers were there with water and snacks every 5k which was most welcome, we would rest at lunchtime under a huge grapevine with large flowers and large shady areas. The locals were very kind and would sit and chat with us and while away the day. We all wore shorts and sun tops but would cover up to respect the locals, the local church bells would ring out noon. We walked through the largest sunflower field which was so colourful and breathtaking. We reached our first 30k stop and stayed in a lovely hotel for the first night, it was great to have a shower and sit down for a meal, time to chat and take it all in and everyone soon got to know each other. We had a nighttime drink and went to bed although it did not seem long before we were up for breakfast and another 30k walk. The sun is shining and that was a good reason to get up, I had my own reason – I was alive, people are all individual and it soon became clear why they had all taken the challenge, all of us were walking to raise funds for someone not just me. I found many that had lost a member of their family to a blood condition or whilst waiting for a bone marrow transplant match, sadly I have known many in my life – I am so lucky to be alive. As we walk I can smell the fresh air and see the sunshine, it is wonderful and makes us feel so healthy.

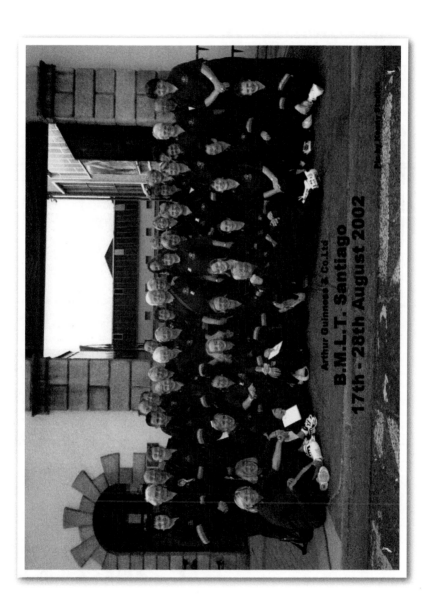

Arthur Guinness & Co.Ltd
B.M.L.T. Santiago
17th - 28th August 2002

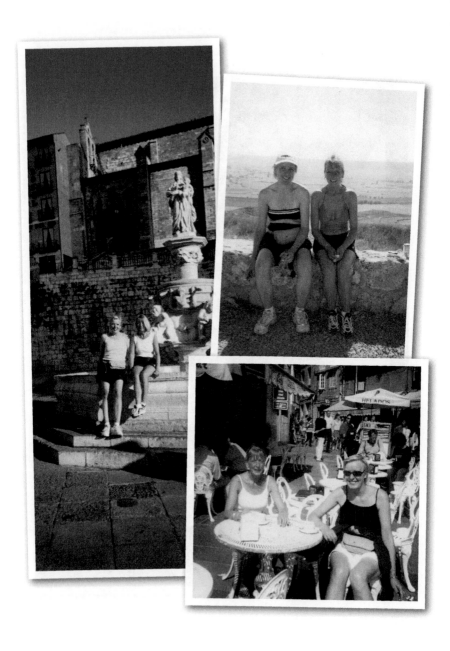

In the days ahead we all started changing colour – no white legs anymore and I reminded everyone to make sure they had sunscreen on. Sun hats were needed as it was getting hotter – 38 degrees in the sunshine. We carried on and every day we would be grateful to achieve our daily goal. The organisers had a video link to record our trip, local radio stations across the land covered the event and I was interviewed and asked to put my appeal out on air, it was sent to America and Ireland to be broadcast over all radio stations.

The pilgrimage walk was fantastic and we celebrated to the end. I took a flight to East Midlands Airport and Annette and the rest of the fundraisers flew back to Eire. When I got home I got many letters congratulating me and saying well done and continue with what you are doing. The newspapers have always followed me and printed my stories and appeals, Radio Leicester's Ben Jackson continues to follow my story and the Anthony Nolan Trust were so pleased and have always thanked me, every penny I raise goes to them and it gives me so much pleasure to give to others.

I have got through 10 years now and arranged a party at the Working Men's Club (of course I made it a fundraiser – £1 to get in, raffles, buffet, karaoke etc). Much to my delight I had a surprise visitor – my nephew Michael who had secretly flown over with Annette, it was fantastic to see him and it turned out to be a super night with loads of dancing and singing and as you can imagine everyone was very happy and having all my family and my friends from Oadby there made the evening even more special – around 200 people came to help me celebrate!

In 2006 I began to feel that I was getting my life back on track and I started to go out at the weekends. I had many friends some of whom were married with children but Tricia and Suzanne would arrange a girlie night out, we are like the golden ladies now, we would dance and sing and have a great buzz when we went out. Every weekend I would shower, hair done, make up in place and I would dress up like a lady. One weekend we went to The Fox in Oadby, I knew everyone in there but I noticed one man aged about 45 with a lovely smile, very handsome – to me he looked like John Thaw. The next weekend we went out again to The Fox and I saw the same man, he smiled at me and as I walked by I said hello. When I came back he introduced himself and said his name was Keith and asked if I would like to go for a drink at some time. That night Keith gave me his telephone number and it was two weeks later that I told myself why not? I was nervous making the call but somehow inside I knew it was going to be a change in my life. Keith picked me up one evening and we went out for a meal, it was a lovely night getting to know each other, I told him all about myself and he told me about his family, he had been married twice before and had two daughters. Both were married Cheryl and Chris had twin boys Tom and Alex and his other daughter Rachel is married to Theo. After our meal we went to the pub, by now we were both at ease, Keith asked if he could see me again and I said yes. The following Sunday we went for a lovely walk at Foxton Locks. Keith is a gentleman, opens doors, walks on the outside of the pavement, would ring me when I am out of work. Keith lived near to where my grandparents lived and knew Tick-Tock Park near Grace Road. At the weekends we would go out and we would often go to the pub that my grandad used to take me to when I was young when grandad would have a bottle of beer and I would enjoy a glass of pop and a packet of crisps. Keith had been living on his own for a long time working as a lorry driver which was long hours and working as a shopfitter sometimes over the water. When I was not working I would go with him – I have now seen many towns and cities that I had not seen before. Wherever we went Keith would work in the shop while I would walk around the town, find a pub for a cheeky half of lager and when it was a hot sunny day I would get an ice cream and sit down and watch the world go by. These were happy times. Keith had a dog called Ben and after work we would take Ben for a walk. We would have cosy nights in and it was not long before I stayed overnight. It soon became every weekend – our time together was growing into love. I started to tidy up the house and did some decorating cheered up the home and Keith appreciated all I had done. We would go to parties and dance the night away, many times we would stagger home – it would be someone celebrating their birthday, when it was in Oadby at either the Oadby Town Football Club or the Rugby Club Keith would bring Ben and stay over. One time we carried home a tray of food for supper as many times there was too much food at parties and my dad would enjoy the supplies. One week Keith said would I like to meet his family, I was nervous as we drove to meet Cheryl, Chris and the twins. We went to Country Park and had a picnic, played games with the twins and I was totally at ease. Cheryl and Chris made me feel very welcome. At a later date I met Theo and Rachel and we met at the local Indian restaurant, again my nerves were in my belly but once again I was at ease. Rachel and Theo now have two children Isabel and Isaac – they call me Granny Alison. We had many days out with all the family and it gave me a good feeling, I could be myself with the children and they were wonderful, it would sit down with all four and read a story, play high and seek, I spy and football – all the things that children should do. Tom and Alex would have sleepovers here and camp in the garden, I had got everything they needed, they would ask when they could do it again and I replied any time you come over here. We would walk to Oadby Tennis Courts in Ellis Park and have lemonade and ice lollies, I felt the children had closed a gap for me, I could not have any children and had delighted in my nieces and nephews but this felt more like a family unit, I always made sure they all had a great time. I have made costumes for their school parties and Halloween – sometimes at what seemed like a moments notice – but it was a joy to see the delight on their faces.

Keith had taken me to Cornwall where I had never been, we went to Padstow and it was lovely. We also took my dad to Cornwall and he loved it. Ben would come everywhere with us – Keith had had him since he was a pup and he was part of the family. Keith and I would talk about our future and how we wanted to live together as it was becoming clear that our love for each other was growing but I didn't want to move from Oadby and I asked Keith if he would like to move in with me and dad. As the bungalow only had one double room, it was decided that we would convert the garage in the garden which was a few feet away from the back door into a room, it was already equipped with electricity and was partially decorated. We spent a lot of time bricking up where the garage doors had been and insulating the property. My neighbour offered me a window as she was having replacement windows installed and before too long we had created a cosy and comfortable double bedroom and Keith and Ben moved in.

In 2009 I planned my next fundraising event – I am now 49 years old and have decided to abseil down the side of the Holiday Inn hotel in Leicester and once again all proceeds go to the Anthony Nolan Trust. It was a perfect day as the sun was shining, family and friends came to support me and once again the media was present in the form of Central News and the Leicester Mercury. The abseil was unnerving, whilst waiting I could not look over the wall as my stomach was churning and it was very scary. I was told "time to go over the wall Alison, just lean back and enjoy". OK I said but my nerves were on edge and I found it tough but I got on with it. One thing that got me through was being aware of the cheers from the car park below

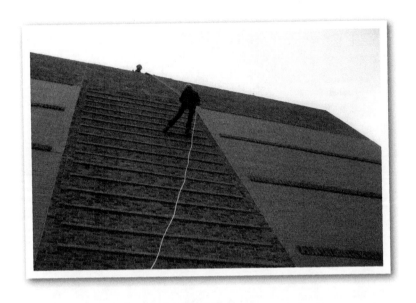

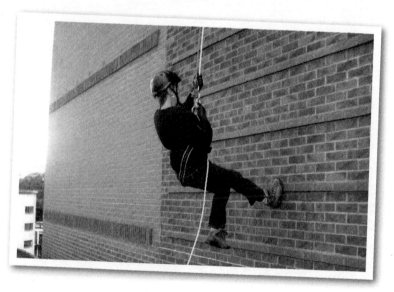

Anthony Nolan Challenge
Holiday Inn 100ft Abseil

Leicester
Saturday 3 October 2009

ENTER ONLINE:
www.anthonynolan.org.uk

The ANTHONY
NOLAN *Trust*
Taking mack lives from leukaemia

46

where everyone had gathered to support me, I made it down and my legs were like jelly but the buzz you get is worth every minute particularly knowing that I have once again been able to help the Anthony Nolan Trust. With this event another £470 was raised. Life was good, I continued to visit the Hammersmith Hospital every year and thanks to Annette it is wonderful to be alive – what can I do next!! Annette and I keep in touch every week and she loves to hear all about the events that I do and she also tells me about what she has done in Eire with her fundraising events as Annette is like me and keen to do everything for everyone.

In 2011 I was due to turn 50 in August so I wanted to celebrate in style – what could my next challenge be? I know I thought – I will do a skydive! I started contacting the press (Leicester Mercury and the Oadby & Wigston News) to advertise my next fundraising venture, they have always been very supportive of me in this respect. I also made contact with my friend Ben Jackson at Radio Leicester. As usual my appeal to raise awareness was put out for young people to join the register and in particular I stressed the need for ethnic groups to join as there is an urgent need for donors for them.

July 2011 has been booked for the tandem skydive. Annette thought I was mad but I knew I still had her support and the full support of all the family no matter what my next venture would involve. I travelled to Langar airfield Nottingham with all the family, it was a lovely sunny day and we sat in deckchairs, picnic baskets out and following a short drill and briefing and being kitted out I waited for my name to be called. I was not nervous and I could not wait to get into the air, I enjoyed watching all the parachutes coming down and landing. Finally my name was called, I was ready but Keith and dad were nervous. I went to the group where the 8 of us were waiting to meet our tandems. My tandem was a young man called Ryan, it was a sign that all would go well as he had a beautiful smile and he was Irish! I asked if we could sit at the back of the plane and when he asked why I replied that once everyone else had gone I would have the sky to myself – his laughter was light. It was so exciting, I waved to everyone and said I will see you soon and we then travelled to the plane by jeep. The sky was clear blue as we boarded and the other people were nervous but I could not stop smiling. I could not wait. The plane was up quickly and we reached 12,000 feet above the clouds, some passengers were getting really nervous but everyone did it for their own reasons. "Are you ready Alison" Ryan asked – couldn't stop smiling, we inched our bums to the doorway and Ryan counted to three and we went on three, the freefall was amazing and in 8 seconds we travelled fastly, my cheeks were bubbled and I kept my mouth closed for fear that my false teeth might fall out! They didn't and then the chute opened and we travelled through the clouds it was amazing, I took the guide ropes and said are you ready Ryan, I pulled on the right rope and we whizzed right which was an experience I could not forget. Suddenly I could see the countryside and little dots on the ground, I was so happy and knew that I had raised great funds for the Anthony Nolan. Landing was great, legs stretched out, we hit the ground safely and Ryan and I had the biggest smiles on our faces. I couldn't get up immediately as my legs felt like jelly but I wanted to get up and do it all over again but this time from a higher height. All my family were watching and had big smiles on their faces. I was greeted by Keith and dad, I was on such a high. They were talking about the fact that they had watched everyone not just me. Langar is a place anyone can go for the day, take a picnic, there is a café and bar and you can simply sit and watch the skydives – it is a lovely day out.

Now my feet are firmly back on the ground, the sky dive had been videoed and I could not wait to receive my copy in the post. I rang Annette and the whole family were delighted. I wanted to celebrate and have a pint or two. The Anthony Nolan were also delighted as I raised £1,200.

Life continued to get better, Summer and Autumn came and went and Christmas was lovely our first one together – Keith, dad and Ben. As a carer I would always work Christmas day so that all the younger staff could have the time off with their children but this year I had said no as I felt it would be wonderful to have our first Christmas living together so I shopped for all the goodies – turkey and all the trimmings, I cooked the ham and made a trifle as Keith and dad love my trifle. I had made the Christmas cake starting in September to ensure that I got it right, I brought all the bits for a family Christmas – After Eight mints, nuts, orange and lemon slices, dates and a bottle of port. Before cooking I would send Keith and dad to the pub, I have already wrapped the presents – chocolate orange, slippers, a new jumper and a bottle of whisky for dad, bottle of single malt whisky, new jumper and a new Tigers rugby shirt for Keith. Keith and I would go to Midnight service on Christmas Eve – time to reflect with everyone and remember all our loved ones. A fabulous first Christmas together!!

In the following September 2012 I fell outside, I could not get up and held on to the dustbins. Keith picked me up and got me inside and told me to lie and rest on the sofa. I always have my medicine bag with me but when I woke up I could not get my words out and had lost my voice. Keith had seen the stoke advertisements on television and said I am taking you to the LRI Alison. We got there quickly and I was asked my date of birth – couldn't remember or speak. I was taken straight in and plugged into the monitors, doctors came and said I had had a stroke. I was told that I would have to have an operation as there was a blood clot on its way to my brain, I was in shock and couldn't speak and had no life in my arms. Keith had stayed by my side throughout the night. Once I was in the stroke ward Keith rang my dad who was also in shock. Keith brought dad down on the Sunday but before they came they had both rung

Annette and various friends. Annette was on the first flight to come and see me, I burst into tears when she came in but the doctors and nurses on the stroke ward were all fabulous, I can't thank them enough. I was prepared to go to surgery and I had seen the blood clot on the monitor. It was bursting to get into my brain and I was still in shock. I was frightened, would I get through this I thought as I was still in shock. I drifted into sleep and I had my operation. Keith, dad and Annette were all there when I woke up, I was worried and the shock was still present. The next week was comfortable, the doctors would see me each morning and the nurses were wonderful but it took a week to get my speech back. The operation had been successful but when the doctors asked me a question, Keith wanted to answer for me but the doctor said no Alison has to do it. Whenever a person is in hospital it is very hard for them lonely sad and worrying – they just want to get home. I need to put it in my mind that I have to be strong. I asked the nurses could I please have a shower, the nurses said of course you can Alison and we will help you. As I still have a weak left side and my arms and legs were affected, I accepted the help. Keith was wonderful, he had been by my side 24/7. He told his family, his daughter Cheryl is a speech therapist and she visited me several times when I got home. I had lots of support on my road to recovery from friends, family and neighbours.

It took a good 6 months to feel better and I have now recovered. My speech is sometimes difficult if I am in a crowd. I have difficulty with conversations as I struggle to get my words out, sometimes I can't use my left arm and have to use my elbow for strength when I am cutting food. I struggle with my spelling when I am texting, my friends laugh as I get the letters all wrong but there is no malice as it is part of my character. I get things wrong quite a lot of the time and sometimes numbers are too much for me, I can't always seem to get them to add up.

TRUST: RAISING FUNDS 20 YEARS SINCE TRANSPLANT

New charity challenge for 'exceptional' Alison

by **ADRIAN TROUGHTON**

Alison Mayes has spent the last two decades raising money for the Anthony Nolan blood cancer charity.

The 49-year-old has supported the charity since she received a life-saving bone marrow transplant from her sister, Annette.

Twenty years ago, Alison was suffering from aplastic anaemia – a condition where the bone marrow does not produce enough cells to replenish blood cells in the body – and was lucky to have a match in her older sibling.

Alison, from Oadby, said: "I was fortunate because Annette was a match for me, but I knew that without her I would have had to turn to the Anthony Nolan charity.

DONORS

"As I lay there recovering, I vowed that if I got fit and well I would do what I could to help them."

Alison has been true to her word since the transplant in 1991, raising £86,000 for the charity.

Over the years, she has climbed Ben Nevis, abseiled down Leicester's Holiday Inn, walked 150km in Spain, organised raffles and staged quizzes to raise the cash.

She has also encouraged more than 40 people to sign up the charity's national register of potential donors.

Alison celebrates her 50th birthday this year and intends to mark it with a special sponsored event. She said: "I have signed up to do a skydive. The thought of me jumping out a plane at 10,000ft is scary, but when I had the transplant I was given a 20 per cent chance of survival, so that was scarier."

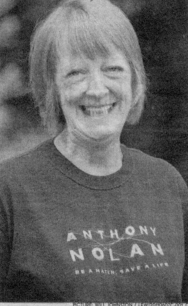

PICTURE: WILL JOHNSTON / LEW120110607C-001_C
DAREDEVIL: Alison Mayes, 49, of Oadby, is doing a skydive to mark 20 years since she had a transplant

Alison makes her leap of faith on July 31, four days before her 50th.

She said: "I am having a big party at the Oadby Legion Club for about 300 people. It is my way of saying thanks for all the years of support."

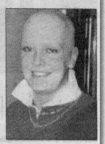

FLASHBACK: Alison, when she was in hospital

Anthony Nolan regional fund-raising assistant Fiona Gaffney said: "We are so impressed by the amount of money that Alison has been able to raise so far, and how much more she has planned.

"As a charity we are always looking to raise funds in order to recruit more donors to our stem cell register, grow our cord blood programme and fund pioneering research into stem cell transplants.

"We couldn't do it without support from exceptional people like Alison."

Anyone who wants to sponsor Alison can call her on 0116 271 8370.

■ To join the Anthony Nolan register, you must be aged between 18 and 40, weigh more than eight stone (51kg) and be in general good health.

For more information, or to apply to join the register, call 0303 303 0303 or visit:

www.anthonynolan.org

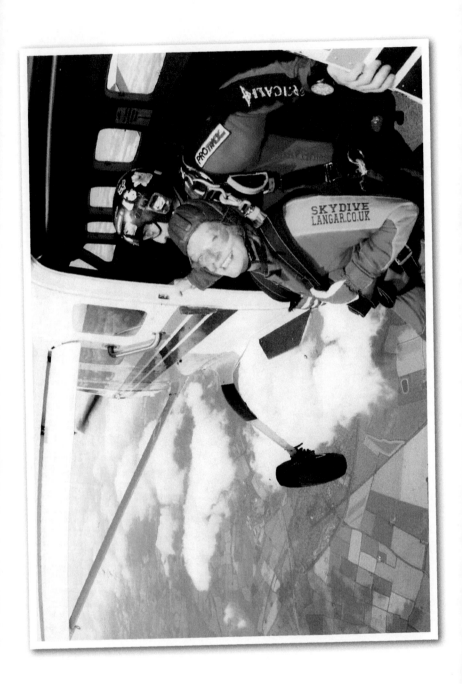

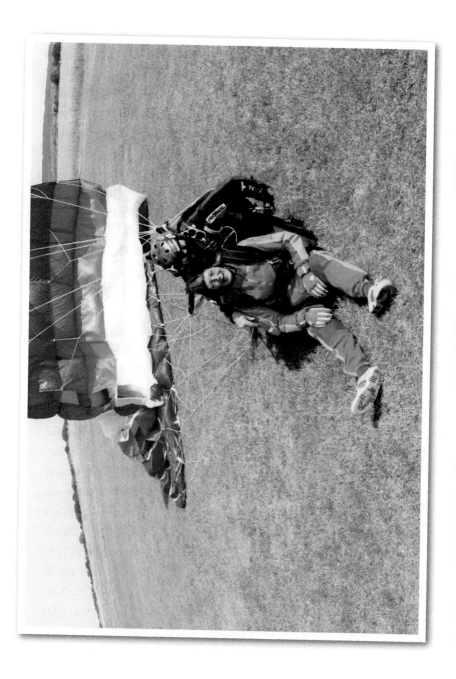

I am back at work now, I appreciate every day I wake up and nothing can worry me again. One day I was at work and I had a message to go down to reception where I was handed a huge bunch of flowers with a card that said "WILL YOU MARRY ME?" I couldn't believe it and thought was it a joke, I was smiling all the way back upstairs I told all the staff and the residents and showed them the flowers and message, I couldn't wait to get home. Keith had asked dad for permission to propose and dad had obviously said yes and the first thing I did when I got home was to tell Keith that my answer was a definite YES! I phoned Annette and soon all the family and friends knew and were delighted for us both. Keith's family were also delighted. I asked him when we could get the ring and he said anytime. We talked for much of the night and the plans started to form, Keith wanted us to get married in church and we went to see the vicar at St Peter's Church, we brought the ring – a beautiful Solaki diamond but Keith decided he did not want a ring. Keith asked if I would like to wear his mother's wedding ring which was an antique but my finger was too small and it would have been expensive to have it altered. I said to him why didn't he wear it and so he did.

There was a busy time ahead but we both loved it, we would sit in the garden with a glass of wine and plan our wedding day, we didn't need any presents so we told everyone there would not be a wedding list as we already had everything between us. When we went to see the vicar she said she had looked me up on Goggle and I asked "What's Google?" which caused much amusement. The church was booked for 14th September 2013. Here I have to tell you about Annette and Jim's daughter Katie my niece. She owns a dress boutique called Katie's Couture selling debutante dresses, ball gowns and wedding dresses. As soon as she could she rang me and asked if she could visit me and of course I said yes so Katie and family came over on the next flight as she had something she wanted to tell me in person. We had a family celebration sitting outside at Weatherspoons as the weather was warm, we had a few pints together and Katie told me that she had something back at home for me in Eire. Katie asked if I would fly over to Eire soon and I insisted she tell me why whereupon she said that she had a wedding gown in the shop which she would not sell as it was to be mine. Katie had kept the dress and dreamt of me, we were all so happy, I said I can't believe it and I could not wait to contact Annette and Jim when I got home. Annette booked my flight for three weeks time. Keith was happy – it was a dream come true.

We wanted a simple wedding and went to see two place for the reception and in the end we booked the Wigston Stage Hotel the cost of which we shared. I chose all pastel colours as the colour scheme. I started saving £100 a week to pay for the church, we had the choir and church bells and we started planning the guest list. Keith's sister Joan and her husband Gordon had been making cakes for a long time and they told us that all Keith's siblings wanted to pay for us to have a three tier wedding cake – one more thing sorted!

Next on my list of things to do was my visit to Katie, Keith took me to the airport and I said see you next week. During the flight I had time to think – who would have thought it, I was going to marry Keith. I had taken an empty suitcase with me to bring back my wedding dress – would it fit me I thought. Annette and Jim met me at the airport and we could not stop smiling. They live near to Kerry Airport in a big bungalow with a lovely sea view on a sunny day but unfortunately it does rain a lot in Kerry! Annette had planned a girlie day and later we all had a wonderful meal all us together, Jim was very happy and excited about our wedding plans. We cracked open a bottle of wine or two during the evening and then it was time to see THE DRESS!! Annette was giddy with excitement, Sarah and Christopher were back home but Katie unfortunately could not be there but Sarah pressed a button on her phone and Katie was there – I think it was Skype but I am not sure – I am a pen and paper girl myself as I don't do Facebook or Twitter etc. I had said to Katie that I wanted a simple fitted dress with a train, slim and elegant. Did I get a big surprise when Annette brought the dress through to her bedroom – I felt overwhelmed – the dress had a long train, it is a fitted dress that ties at the back, a sweetheart neckline, sequins on the bodice. I stepped into it and it fitted like a glove! Annette and Sarah were helping me and Katie was watching on Skype. Annette pulled the ribbons tight and I had a super elegant dress, I couldn't believe it, I was so happy and a few tears flowed as I thought about my mum Mo and how she would have loved to see this. I said it is going to be tough without mum as she would have loved to be with me. Tears gone and Annette popped a bottle of "fizz" as I shouted a triumphant "IT FITS"!! Before we joined Jim and Chris Annette said I have something else to show you – Katie had organised dresses for my bridesmaids – Isabel, Keith's granddaughter, had a white dress that would make her look like a fairy princess and Michaela's dress was pastel pink with a sash, they were both beautiful. I suggested to Annette that we could use the sash on Michaela's dress to make a bow for Isabel's dress. You recall I said I had brought an empty suitcase to take my wedding dress home – I have a bigger case now! Katie and the family said the gowns would be their wedding gift – I had to phone Keith straightaway and tell him and he was as thrilled as I was. We agreed that the plans were now really coming together – the church was booked, the reception venue was booked, my wedding dress and the bridesmaids' dresses were ready, the cake was sorted and Keith told me that he had asked Graham to be his best man – I felt we were really on our way.

Keith picked me up from the airport and as soon as I returned home I put the precious dresses in the small lounge room and banned anyone from going in there. We later collected Michaela so that she could try her bridesmaid's dress on as we had an appointment with the dressmakers who was to make the sash for Isabel's dress and also shorten my dress and when I had to go back to collect my dress I asked Tricia and Suzanne to come with me as I wanted them to see my dress. We had tears and hugs and it was all very overwhelming. Tricia and Suzanne are my closest friends and we have many years of memories together, they also knew I would be sad as mum would not be there. I asked Tricia to be with me on the day to help me dress and get ready. Keith and I sat together one evening and agreed that we could accommodate all our guests. Keith, Graham, Michael, dad, Tom and Alex were booked in for their suits (we had already decided no tails) and pastel colours for ties etc were chosen to match the bridesmaids dresses. Keith asked where I would like to go for our honeymoon and I said how about Majorca. We had been once together but I had been twice – the first time when I took "John Smith" over! I started to pay monthly towards the flowers at Tippetts in Oadby, the ladies there knew me well and asked me if I had a photo of mum that they could incorporate into my bouquet – I thought that was a lovely sentiment as it meant I could carry mum with me on my wedding day. I went home and found a photo of mum taken on Banner beach and took it back to Tippetts. I told Keith about this and he was as happy as I was.

A friend at work said she wanted to do the flowers for the church and the reception and I said that would be wonderful and offered to pay. She said no, this was to be a gift from everyone at work, what a lovely gift. Everything was falling into place and it felt wonderful.

Keith took me to get the wedding ring – I felt so proud that I had got everything from Oadby my home town where I had been born and still lived. The only thing to be organised was the vintage open topped car with red leather seats that I really wanted as my wedding car. We also picked up all the mens' suits together with their shiny shoes. We then went to the Wigston Stage to pay the balance on the reception venue. The wedding organisers were great and very helpful and it was going to be everything that we wanted. Hen night and stag party were planned!

Keith moved out the Wednesday before the wedding on the 14th as various family members were starting to arrive and some of the girls were due to stay with me at the bungalow following my hen night. On 12th September I had my hen night, Jim and dad went to meet Keith and the other blokes as the house was full of ladies. The hen night was a hoot, we practically took over Weatherspoons, there must have been 30 or more of us there, I took it steady but still had a fabulous time, we were all so happy. On the Friday we went out for lunch and we talked about how I thought I would never marry, I can't believe that since my transplant my life has just got better every day and tomorrow I would be getting married. My neighbours came round with gifts and wished me a lovely day for tomorrow. We all had a relaxing night and I was thrilled to have all the family with me – it was magical! I went to bed at midnight but made sure all the girls bunked down on the lounge floor were OK.

Saturday 14th September 2013 –THE BIG DAY!

I was up early and was greeted by dad and the girls. We had breakfast and a cup of tea – just like any other day until I suddenly realised it was my wedding day! I had showered and the hairdresser and my make-up artist arrived, the kitchen was full of bustle and joy, so surreal I had to pinch myself. Tricia, Michelle and Michaela arrived, Annette helped Michaela to dress and then Michaela had her hair done. I had arranged for Annette, Katie and Sarah to have their hair done at the hairdressers that morning as a surprise and Katie and Sarah had ringlets in their hair and looked beautiful. We popped a bottle of bubbly. The flowers arrived and I saw my bouquet – freesias and carnations in my chosen pastel colours but what made it extra special was seeing my mum's photo within the bouquet and I had a lump in my throat. I had ordered buttonholes for all the men and a special corsage for Annette. Dad was happy and proud but as you can appreciate with all us girls around, it was difficult for him to get into the bathroom! Michaela loved her dress and Michelle was in awe seeing us all look so beautiful. Tom, Alex and Isabel arrived from the Wigston Stage where they had been staying, they were all dressed and ready. I asked them if they would carry my train and they were very excited to do so. It was going to be an awesome day but I was getting nervous, butterflies in my stomach. I was whisked away to my bedroom to get dressed with Annette, Sarah, Katie and Tricia attending to dress me. Before I knew it the photographer had arrived, it was all crazy but everyone was still smiling! After having photographs taken in the garden, Tom and Alex announced that the car had arrived but it did not have red leather seats! Keith had asked them to keep it a secret as it was a surprise – he had ordered a yellow open topped Rolls Royce! Everyone then left for the church – just me, dad and Sarah remained – our time at last.

When the car returned I said to dad shall we go? It was 2.10 and the sun was shining brightly, I was driven through the village to the church and everyone was out to see me, waving and smiling. It was as we arrived that I became a little teary, there were so many people waiting to see me arrive, I walked up to the church and I saw Tom, Alex, Isabel and Michaela, Tricia was there to touch up my lipstick which I knew my mum would have done if she could have been there. Tom and Alex were so excited and as I turned around and Alex gave me a nudge and a wink – I will never forget that. Dad and I started to walk down the aisle and I could not believe how packed the church was, Keith turned around and looked at me, I was nervous. We had chosen "Morning has broken" as the first hymn and the choir and congregation really sang out. The ceremony began, I was lost for words as the vicar greeted everyone and talked about me. I began to struggle but felt so happy, Rachel handed me a handkerchief, I was glad to sit down as my legs felt like jelly. We said our vows and sang "All things bright and beautiful". Tricia and Graham were our witnesses when we signed the register. We were married – I am now Mrs Alison Shatford!

We walked out of the church and everyone was happy, it was such a beautiful day. Half of Oadby seemed to be there, former teachers, neighbours, work colleagues it was amazing and the church bells were ringing. Photos galore were taken and finally we managed to get into the car, we drove through the village – people waving, cars hooting – it was absolutely amazing. We then drove to Knighton Park to have more photos taken (and to have a quick cigarette!)

Time to get everyone to the Wigston Stage which fortunately is not that far to travel. When we arrived Tricia was there to touch up my lipstick and put my wedding bag on the table. Everyone clapped and cheered as the Master of Ceremonies said "Please be upstanding for Mr and Mrs Shatford". The venue looked gorgeous with all the pastel colours, the dance floor was lit up and there was a big screen behind it with our names on. We were asked by the photographer to have pictures taken. The wedding breakfast was amazing and the three tier wedding cake was incredible – all of our guests gathered round as we cut the cake – I bet you can't guess which cake went first – OK you're right – the yummy chocolate one! When we sat at our table the view was outstanding, all our family and friends in front of us, all wearing lovely bright colours and smiling and on our table my bouquet with my mum's picture. The tables were all adorned with flowers and candles and the sun was constantly shining through the windows. Perfect! I looked over at dad and he was smiling and obviously very proud and happy.

Our day had been perfect and as we started our wedding breakfast I said thank you to my husband. We had been blessed by our families – all the assistance with the dresses, cakes etc. The speeches were fantastic, Keith's speech made us laugh and cry – he is such a gentleman. We had gifts for the bridesmaids, best man and usher and I had a special gift for Annette because without her I might never have had this fantastic day, we have a very special bond that will never go away. Keith and I both needed the loo and we were able to have a moment to ourselves – we toasted each other with champagne and had a cigarette (naughty I know but after all it was OUR wedding day).

At 6.00 p.m. the room as altered to a disco. Other guests arrived to join us for the evening. I said all I wanted at that stage was a pint outside as it was a beautiful evening. My dear friend Paul overheard my request and got us both a pint and sat outside with me as we drank. Guests were still arriving, the whole atmosphere was amazing. Once I went back inside Keith and I were called up to start the dancing – our first dance as husband and wife – it was Whitney Houston "I will always love you" – very appropriate. A buffet was laid on and guess what – a second chocolate cake appeared which went down just as well as the first! The evening progressed well and it was 2.00 a.m. before we retired but even then we spent time reflecting on what a perfect day we had had.

Many of our guests were staying over and we joined them for breakfast the next morning. Everyone was still happy from the day before, it had been perfect in every way and everyone had enjoyed it. We decided we would stay an extra night until the Monday. Later when everyone had left we collected our presents and took them to our room, we were absolutely amazed as we had said no presents – obviously nobody had taken note of this – we had lovely presents and we spent time enjoying reading the accompanying cards. I had even received letters from my GP and cards from the hospitals. Later that day we went out for lunch and visited dad, he was happy to see us as indeed was Ben, dad gave us our gift (which we banked on the Monday!) Keith's family had joined in to buy us new garden furniture which was wonderful, we were feeling very overwhelmed. We left and went out for the rest of the day and returned to the Wigston Stage for the evening.

On Monday we went home and on the Tuesday we flew to Majorca for two weeks. The people at the hotel knew us and we had further celebrations with them which was wonderful. We had time to reflect over our wedding, the build up to our wedding was like a dream but now my dream is reality – I am Mrs Shatford, Keith had married me for who I was with no airs and graces, our love was strong, over the years it has grown stronger and stronger.

—

I had spent 23 years doing care work which I enjoyed but I had reached a stage in my life when I felt I needed to have a job that was nine to five. I asked in the shops round Oadby if they were looking for any staff and I walked into Oadby DIY – I could not believe it, I got an interview and started working there three weeks later. I loved the job, Oadby DIY was also a garden centre and I love gardening, I soon got to know the customers and was fairly knowledgeable about DIY having done most of my DIY when I was at the flat at Brabazon Road where I re-vamped the bathroom changing the suite and the kitchen, decorating etc. When we moved to the bungalow there was not really anything to do as it was perfect.

In March 2016 I decided to get a dog as a gentleman had come into the shop and asked if it would be alright to bring his dog in, I said what breed of dog is it and he said "A Maltese". I looked over the counter I saw a small dog with melting eyes, he was clear white with a curved fluffy tail – I was totally smitten. I telephoned the RSPCA to ask if they knew any breeders local to the area and they gave me the number of a lady called Sue who had been breeding champions for some time, she lived out at Melton Mowbray and I contacted her that evening. I asked if she had any male puppies available and she said she would call me back as some puppies were being born as we spoke. She rang me back and said "I have five females and one male in this litter", I immediately asked if she would keep the male for me. In my mind I knew that Keith's dog Ben was getting older, I had spent many hours on my own while Keith was out with Ben – there were a couple of reasons why I wanted to get a dog because it would be company for dad while we were out working and also because Ben was getting older. Unfortunately on 5th February 2018 we lost Ben, he was 17 years old and had been everywhere with Keith since he was a puppy even accompanying Keith when he was out lorry driving. We both took Ben to the vets although it was too painful for Keith to stay in the surgery so I told him to go for a walk. I held Ben until the injection took effect. Ben knew us but would not allow anyone else near, but that was him – so special.

In May 2017 Keith and I both left Oadby DIY – it was not the same once new owners took over. Later we were relaxing in the garden with our friends Celia and Lee and I started to think about my life, I felt I had done all I could but there was still something missing so I asked them all could I work in a charity shop. Keith said but you have your own charity so why not open your own charity shop for the Anthony Nolan Trust. We all asked what she would call the shop and Lee jokingly said how about "Alison's

Bits and Bobs" – and we fell in love with the idea. I started to look for a vacant shop in the Oadby and Wigston area but the rates were too high. I tried looking on line and we would drive around at weekends looking for empty shops. It was a stressful time. I met up with Celia for a drink after work one evening and as we sat outside the Weatherspoons a rainbow appeared in the sky and Celia said "that's an omen – you will find a shop soon". Keith had spotted a vacant premises on Welford Road and we went to view the shop, the landlord was a lovely man and from the start I knew it would be the shop for me. I noticed the side road was called Ashford Road and I felt that was another omen that I should take the shop – Ashford – Shatford, it seemed like fate. We went to sign the paperwork in the evening and went to collect the keys on 3rd August 2017. We started to paint the outside of the shop – the window frames were green but I wanted pure white with a pillar box red front door!

It was now time to start setting things up properly – Celia works for a bank and was a great help, and agreed to be a director of the company and assisted us when Keith and I opened the business account. I have never owned my own business before and the bank were great and pointed me in the right direction to get started. Annette, Jim and all the family were so pleased for me and the Oadby community wished me well. I had everyone offering to help and soon the donations of clothing and bits and bobs were pouring in.

Celia asked her friend Raj if he would be able to help design the boards for outside the shop, they look wonderful and to this day I can't say how much I appreciate it. We set a date for opening the shop – 19th August 2017 – my shop was full, donations kept coming in, it was amazing the generosity of people I know and those I had not met before.

Opening day finally arrived – family, friends and members of the public attended together with the Leicester Mercury and my friend Ben Jackson from Radio Leicester was also there. It was a marvellous day and the atmosphere on Welford Road was exhilarating.

I do miss Charlie when I am at work (although he has been to the shop a couple of times). When I get home I take him out for a walk and then we come home and it is playtime. He has a lovely character and plays with all the other dogs large or small – I recall Keith and I took him to Foxton Locks one day and stopped for a pint – when Keith came out with the drinks Charlie was playing with a large Rottweiller who was sitting down so that Charlie could play with him, it made a wonderful picture. I have a picture of Charlie in the shop and many people ask me about him. I have made my shop welcoming, the students come in regularly from Leicester University and they come from all parts of the world, the young ladies want to learn how to cook and I have given them some of my mum's recipes for simple cakes, meals etc. I tell them about the history of Leicester – Richard III, Bradgate Park and Old John, our famous sons the Attenborough brothers, Gary Lineker, the Space Centre and the museums. The shop is a wonderful place and the people who come in look through my folder about my bone marrow transplant and ask many questions about it so I explain about my life and how lucky I am. I have a warm connection with customers and the children love to come in – I have a kiddies corner set aside for them where they can play with some of the toys and games. I always have a small treat for them and mums and dads say they can't walk past without the children wanting to come in and see me.

Now perhaps you can see why my shop is so important to me, I have the unending support of my family, friends, the general public and the media. Without that support I would not have been able to make regular donations to the Anthony Nolan

Trust. I have had to take a lot of medications since my transplant and my stroke, years ago I had to take 50 tablets a day round the clock, now I am down to 7 and only one relates to my transplant! I will take penicillin for life and have to take Vitamin D daily, my life has been a sometimes arduous journey but I am still here to tell the tale.

I wanted to thank everyone who knows me – family, friends, the dedication from the hospitals and the staff and all of the Oadby community. I cannot obviously name all the friends who are so dear to me but you all know who you are. I love you all and I particularly want to thank the public who support me every day in my shop. I am here to help anyone I can and to listen, anyone who is facing the daunting prospect of a transplant I wish you and your loved ones well. I give you my love and strength to get you through. I am here for anyone who wants to know about the bone marrow register or to talk about treatments. I will always support the Anthony Nolan Trust by continuing to raise awareness and regular donations. I know that every day someone somewhere is going to be diagnosed with a blood disorder, I am here for anyone who is watching over a loved one going through this, I have learnt and seen at first hand that the people closest to you suffer as well and may I say don't compare yourself to someone else, you are an individual, let the warm tears fall on your cheeks – do not be afraid to cry you are after all only human. I spent many years crying to myself but know now that it is ok to cry but try to smile instead, the sun will shine again soon. Take every day as a blessing, when you wake up it is a new day and you need to live it to the full, don't look back as it is the future that counts. Love each other and hug each other and be happy, share your feelings and don't let things get you down. If my book accomplishes one thing it will be to give people hope and for that I will be happy.

I must make a special mention of a little girl called Molly. When her and her mum came into the shop we started talking about the Anthony Nolan Trust and she told me that Molly had had to have chemotherapy and she had been in hospital with leukemia. Molly has three sisters and one had been approved as a bone marrow donor. Moly had weekly visits to the LRI and every week they would come into the shop to visit me. It wasn't long before the whole family came, they knew they had somewhere to go for courage and comfort, a smile and a dance and we would turn the radio up, it was a complete joy to see such a wonderful family and all the happy faces when they were here. I did ask Molly if I could include her in my book and the big smile on her face told me that it would be ok! It is now 15 months later and Molly is in remission and doing so well, her appointments at the LRI are now every two months. I have seen all four girls growing up which has been a joy to witness.

Thank you all for reading my story, life is for living and I am proof of that, if life is getting you down a bit put the radio on as music is a good source for lifting your spirits.

I must send much love and thanks to Keith my husband who has supported me and taken care of me since he met me. Love and thanks to my dad who took me under his wing since I was 13 and of course my most special thanks to my sister Annette. I will never be able to put into words what you mean to me, it is the hardest thing to write, I love all the family whether near or far, thank you for being my sister and my friend, we have had many ups and downs over the years but we always get through it don't we! If it was not for you Annette who gave me the generous gift of life, I would not be here today to share my story, you are a million stars and always will be to me, I love you!

St Peter's Church Oadby

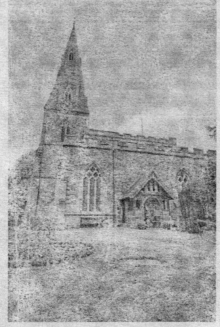

The Marriage of

Alison Eunice Mayes to Keith Shatford

Saturday 14th September 2013

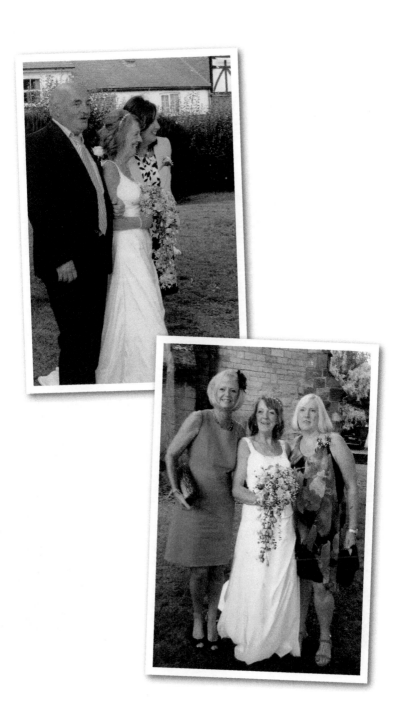

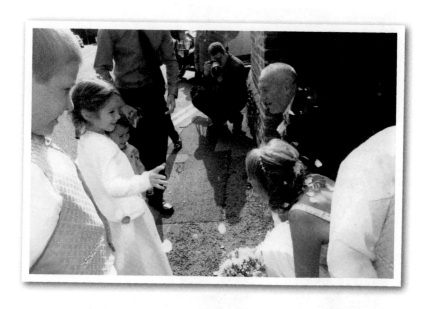

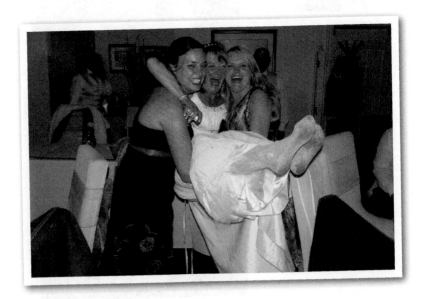

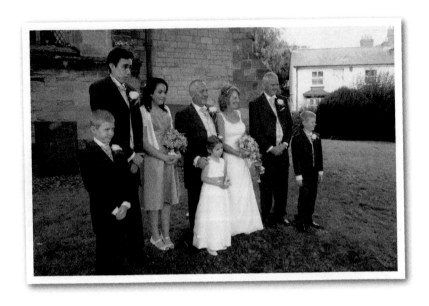

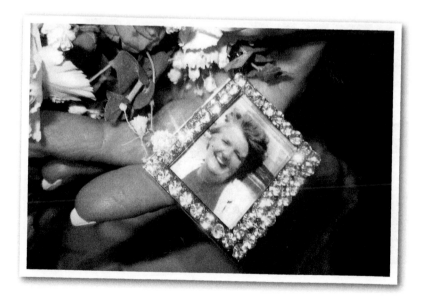

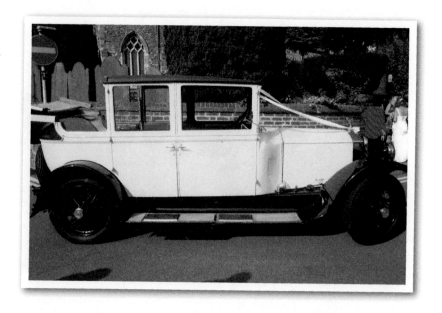

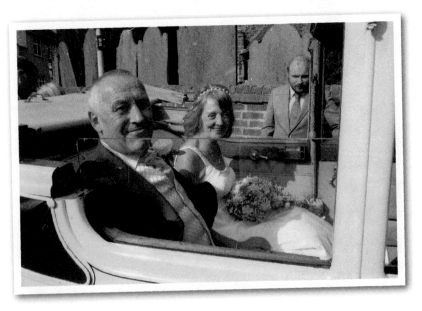

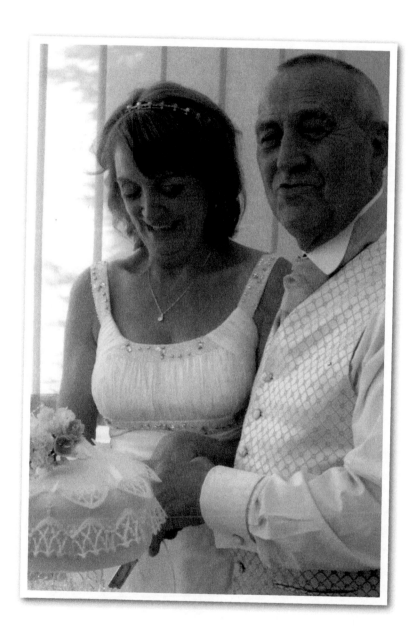

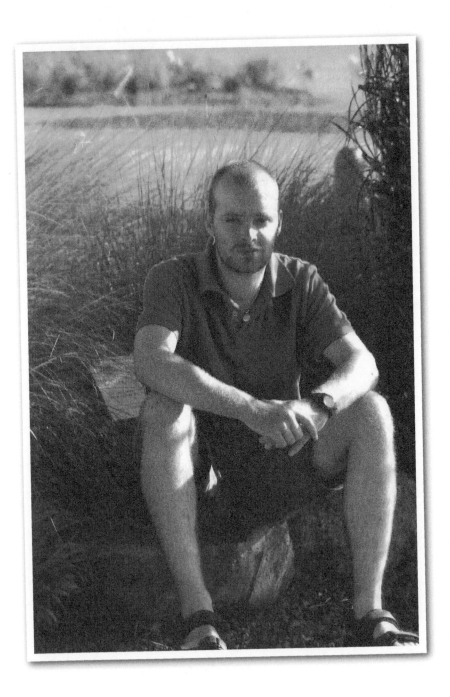

Nana

A warm hearted women with charm and effect,
she changed all the people that ever once she met.
A heart of gold pure and through,
A brillant mind that shone right through,
A winning smile that broke our hearts,
That we were ever broken apart.

I loved her more than words can say
We mourn the loss every day,
No matter what we'll not forget,
The memorys that we cherish best.
In my heart I keep her close,
And in my mind I keep a note,
Of all the good times we spent together,
They themselves will live forever.

Her sense of humour was the best,
When others were down she would not be depressed.
She laughed at the world and dealt to it joy,
From good to the bad whatever she had .
Never did I hear her complain,
What life had to throw no one better did know.
But she was a women who liked to embrace,
Hit the world head on with a forward face.
  In my heart I keep you strong and there you are forever long ,
  and I hope to see you again one day, thats the one
       Thing I pray

For you Nana

ALISON

Many years ago I stopped writing poetry & told Myself
I'd never write any again

    But this was one for the road , I'd like you
    to have it,
because , Mo was all of these things & a paticulary special
    lady

luv
Chris.

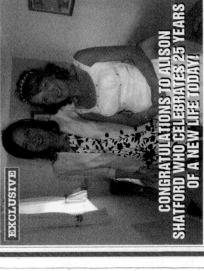

THE NATION REJOICES AS ALISON CELEBRATES 25 YEARS OF LIFE! P2,3,4,5,6 & 7

THE News

18 Nov 2016

25 TODAY

EXCLUSIVE

CONGRATULATIONS TO ALISON SHATFORD WHO CELEBRATES 25 YEARS OF A NEW LIFE TODAY!

FIGHTER ALISON SHATFORD. Celebrating in New Zealand is her niece Sarah O'Donnell, who said, "Ali is a tough cookie, and I am very lucky to have such a strong, sexy, beautiful lady to call my Auntyi".

BIG CONGRATULATIONS AND BEST WISHES FOR THE NEXT 25 YEARS GORGEOUS.X.

THE News

© Moonpig.com

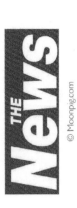

AL,

CONGRATULATIONS ON 25 YEARS!

LOVE YOU SO SO MUCH!
SARAH.X.

WISHING YOU A LOVELY DAY!
I WISH I COULD BE THERE TO GIVE YOU 25 OF THE BIGGEST HUGS!

SO HAPPY THAT YOU ARE CELEBRATING THIS AMAZING DAY!

I AM VERY GRATEFUL FOR YOU!

"DIFFICULT ROADS OFTEN LEAD TO BEAUTIFUL DESTINATIONS".

I HOPE THE LAST 25 YEARS OF DESTINATIONS HAVE BEEN GREAT ONES AND THAT THE NEXT 25 ARE EVEN BETTER!!

LOVE YOU MORE THAN WORDS CAN EXPRESS!
XOXOXOXOXOX

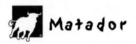 Matador

For exclusive discounts on Matador titles,
sign up to our occasional newsletter at
troubador.co.uk/bookshop